Animal Biotechnology

— Vaccines and Diagnostics —

Markets and Investment Opportunities

The Authors

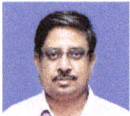

G. Dhinakar Raj is the Project Director of TRPVB and Professor of Tamil Nadu Veterinary and Animal Sciences University, Chennai, with extensive experience in the field of veterinary diagnostics and vaccines. He has more than 26 years of academic and research experience. He has 190 publications to his credit and has developed and commercialized several technologies for field use. He has won several awards including the National Biosciences Award and is the first veterinarian to be awarded the coveted TATA innovation fellowship.

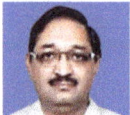

S.R. Rao, Ph. D is Advisor, Department of Biotechnology (DBT), Ministry of Science & Technology; Government of India. He served in various positions in department since 1989 and was associated with implementation of several national level programmes on R&D, technology development and commercialization of biotechnology. Currently, his main responsibility is regulation of genetically engineering products including biosafety and biosecurity. He also specializes in core and cross-sectoral policy issues of Biotechnology policy, development, regulation, safety, public private partnership, international relations and biotech R&D Innovation and Development, and public concerns and consensus building.

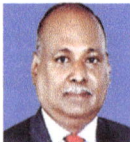

S. Thilagar is presently the Vice-Chancellor of the Tamil Nadu Veterinary and Animal Sciences University, Chennai. He is a renowned small animal surgeon and clinician in this country. He has international work experience as visiting Professor in University Putra Malaysia (2003–2008). He also served as Dean, Rajiv Gandhi Institute of Veterinary Education and Research (Formerly Rajiv Gandhi College of Veterinary and Animal Sciences), Puducherry 2011–2014) and Controller of Examinations at TANUVAS (2010 – 2011). He has published more than 100 research articles both in national and international journals and authored 4 books. He has been the recipient of several State and National awards such as the Best Teacher Award of TANUVAS (1997), Tamil Nadu Scientist Award (1990), Dr. Ratan Singh Memorial Award (2015) *etc.*, to name a few. He has implemented 15 external research projects and is the Chairman/Member of various State Committees.

Animal Biotechnology
— Vaccines and Diagnostics —
Markets and Investment Opportunities

— *Authors* —

G. Dhinakar Raj

S.R. Rao

S. Thilagar

2017

Daya Publishing House®

A Division of

Astral International Pvt. Ltd.

New Delhi–110 002

ISBN: 978-93-86071-68-2 (International Edition)

Publisher's Note:

Published by   :   **Daya Publishing House**®
                                   A Division of
                                   Astral International Pvt. Ltd.
                                   – ISO 9001:2015 Certified Company –
                                   4736/23, Ansari Road, Darya Ganj
                                   New Delhi-110 002
                                   Ph. 011-43549197, 23278134
                                   E-mail: info@astralint.com
                                   Website: www.astralint.com

Digitally Printed at   :   Replika Press Pvt. Ltd.

Abbreviations

AI	Avian Influenza
AN	Andaman and Nicobar Islands
AP	Andhra Pradesh
AR	Arunachal Pradesh
AS	Assam
AT	Anthrax
ABC	Animal Birth Control
ASCAD	Assistance to States for Control of Animal Diseases
BQ	Black Quarter
BR	Bihar
BSL	Biosafety Level
BT	Bluetongue
CAGR	Compound Annual Growth Rate
CCPP	Contagious Caprine Pleuro Pneumonia
CDSCO	Central Drugs Standard Control Organization
CG	Chhattisgarh

CH	Chandigarh
CPV	Canine Parvo Virus
CSF	Classical Swine Fever
CBPP	Contagious Bovine Pleuro Pneumonia
cGMP	Current Good Manufacturing Practices
CFSPH	Center for Food Security and Public Health
CPCSEA	Committee for the Purpose of Control and Supervision of Experiments on Animals
CBD	Convention on Biological Diversity
CRO	Contract Research Organizations
DIVA	Differentiating Infected from Vaccinated Animals
DH	Dadra and Nagar Haveli
DL	Delhi
DAHDF	Department of Animal Husbandry Dairying and Fisheries
DBT	Department of Biotechnology
DD	Daman and Diu
DCGI	Drug Controller General of India
DDMA	District Disaster Management Authority
DBT	Department of Biotechnology
DNA	Deoxyribo Nucleic Acid
ET	Enterotoxaemia
EEC	European Economic Community
ELISA	Enzyme Linked Immunosorbant Assay
FMDCP	FMD Control Program
FSSAI	Food Safety and Standards Authority of India
FMD	Foot and Mouth Disease
FAOSTAT	Statistics Division of FAO
GA	Goa
GADVASU	Guru Angad Dev Veterinary and Animal Sciences University
GCP	Good Clinical Practice
GJ	Gujarat
GLP	Good Laboratory Practices

GoI	Government of India
GIS	**Geographic Information System**
HS	Hemorrhagic Septicemia
HVT	Turkey Herpes virus
HR	Haryana
HP	Himachal Pradesh
IBR	Indian Boilers Regulation
ICAR	Indian Council of Agricultural Research
IIL	Indian Immunologicals Limited
IVRI	Indian Veterinary Research Institute
INR	Indian National Rupee
IBD	Infectious Bursal Disease
IAEC	Institutional Animal Ethics Committee
ILRI	International Livestock Research Institute
IFAH	International Federation of Animal Health
IPPC	International Plant Protection Convention
IB	Infectious bronchitis
IBD	Infectious Bursal Disease
JH	Jharkhand
JK	Jammu and Kashmir
JV	Joint Venture
KL	Kerala
KA	Karnataka
LAMP	Loop Medicated Isothermal Amplification
MP	Madhya Pradesh
MH	Maharashtra
MZ	Mizoram
M and A	Merger and Acquisition
MNC	Multi-National Companies
ML	Meghalaya
MN	Manipur

MSP	Minimum standard protocol
MoHFW	Ministry of Health and Family Welfare
ND	Newcastle Disease
NDMA	National Disaster Management Authority
NEC	National Executive Committee
NIDM	National Institute of Disaster Management
NOC	No Objection Certificate
NIVEDI	National Institute of Veterinary Epidemiology and Disease Informatics
NPRE	National Project for Rinderpest Eradication
NDDB	National Dairy Development Board
NIAB	National Institute of Animal Biotechnology
NIHSAD	National Institute of High Security Animal Diseases
NL	Nagaland
OIE	Office International des Epizooties
OR	Orissa
PB	Punjab
PPF	Policy Perspectives Foundation
PDP	Project Directorate on Poultry
PE	Private Equity
POCT	Point of Care Testing
PY	Pondicherry
PDDSL	Poultry Disease Diagnosis and Surveillance Laboratory
PDFMD	Project Directorate on Foot and Mouth Disease
PCR	Polymerase Chain Reaction
PPR	Peste Des Petits Ruminants
ROI	Return on Investment
RFID	Radio-frequency identification
RJ	Rajasthan
SK	Sikkim
SP/GP	Sheep Pox/Goat Pox
SDMA	State Disaster Management Authority

SEC	State Executive Committee
TB	Tuberculosis
TRPVB	Translational Research Platform for Veterinary Biologicals
TR	Tripura
TANUVAS	Tamil Nadu Veterinary and Animal Sciences University
TN	Tamil Nadu
ULBDMC	Urban Local Body Disaster Management Committee
UK	Uttarakhand
VMP	Veterinary Medicinal Products
VDMC	Village Disaster Management Committee
WHO	World Health Organization
WB	West Bengal

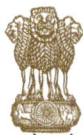

सत्यमेव जयते

कं. विजयराघवन
K. VijayRaghavan

सचिव
भारत सरकार
विज्ञान और प्रौद्योगिकी मंत्रालय
बायोटेक्नोलॉजी विभाग
ब्लाक-2, 7 वां तल, सी. जी. ओ. कम्पलेक्स
लोदी रोड़, नई दिल्ली - 110003

SECRETARY
GOVERNMENT OF INDIA
MINISTRY OF SCIENCE & TECHNOLOGY
DEPARTMENT OF BIOTECHNOLOGY
Block-2, 7th Floor C.G.O. Complex
Lodi Road, New Delhi-110003

Foreword

The livestock sector provides us with meat, dairy and eggs, as well as wool and leather. The importance of livestock farming in Indian agriculture sector has been increasing over the past decade. To maintain livestock health, preventive vaccination and early diagnosis leading to control of diseases should be the hallmark. For a large country like India, the number of veterinary biological manufacturers especially in private sector is very few. Further the dynamics of the multispecies veterinary sector is more challenging than the human medical industry. While most of the vaccines against large animal disease depend on government funded control programmes, poultry is a highly closed and integrated sector and canine market is driven by retail sales and primarily by imports.

A comprehensive updated analysis of markets in livestock industry of India is not available or well documented. Such an analysis will help assess investment opportunities so that the new and profitable start-ups and entrepreneurship are promoted. Such an elaborate review through systematic survey, analysis of information and future projections has been presented in this book. The task has been possible through a DBT-funded project to the Translational Research Platform for Veterinary Biologicals (TRPVB) established in partnership program between DBT and the Tamil Nadu Veterinary and Animal Sciences University (TANUVAS) TRPVB's mandate is to foster 'productization' in the field of veterinary biologicals by converging the presently distant academic research , industry and pathways of regulatory compliance. One of its goals is "to collect and collate available information in the field of veterinary biologicals and serve as a knowledge resource centre for industry, institutions and policy makers". True to its goals, this book is valuable contribution of this platform for use by all stakeholders in promoting growth and investment in livestock sector.

The overall assessment indicates that there is a paradigm shift occurring in this sector through higher investment both by Government and private players with the emergence of new markets, organised farming systems, research and innovation coupled its favourble government policies. The study also identifies gaps for future work on modernising infrastructure in all areas from discovery to markets through strategic investments, reforms in regulations and development of India-specific products to ensure affordability and access to technology for increased profits by livestock farmers.

I would like to heartily congratulate all team members led by Dr. Dhinakar Raj, Project Director, TRPVB and Dr. S.R. Rao, Advisor in DBT in the preparation of this book and also M/s. Sathguru Management Consultants Pvt. Ltd., Hyderabad who has complemented information through their consultancy and the publishers.

(K. VijayRaghavan)

Preface

Livestock is the best insurance against natural calamities such as flood, drought *etc.* in agriculture system of India. Indian livestock sector is one of the largest in the world with a generated output worth Rs. 2075 billions in 2010-11 that comprised 4 per cent of GDP and 26 per cent of the agricultural GDP. Distribution of livestock sector is more equitable than that of land. The importance of livestock sector is growing exponentially. Animal husbandry activities also promote gender equality wherein 90 per cent of employment in livestock sector is shared by women.

In terms of livestock health, vaccines and diagnostics are two sides of the coin of immunoprophylaxis. Prevention is better than cure in the maintenance of livestock health. It is difficult to afford the treatment costs thereby making prophylaxis a better investment. There has been no comprehensive effort to document the status of veterinary vaccines and diagnostics in the country. This lacuna was immediately identified by the Department of Biotechnology, Ministry of Science and Technology, Government of India who funded a project on "Status of Animal biotechnology markets and investment opportunities with special reference to Vaccines and Diagnostics in India" to the Translational Research Platform for Veterinary Biologicals (TRPVB) at the Tamil Nadu Veterinary and Animal Sciences University (TANUVAS), Chennai.

TANUVAS is a premiere and the first dedicated veterinary university in India and its contribution to field of veterinary vaccines and diagnostics has been immense. It has made a pioneering attempt in documenting the status of veterinary vaccines and diagnostics industry in India. To complement this effort TRPVB hired the consultancy of M/s. Sathguru Management Consultants Private Limited, Hyderabad who was also instrumental in collecting information and analysis. Coupled with their information, TRPVB has complemented with additional data along with other inputs in related areas through their knowledge and expertise.

In addition to the vaccines and diagnostics other areas highlighting regulations, biosafety, animal quarantine, economic impact of diseases *etc.* have also been compiled. All these areas pertinently complement the animal industry in this country. We strongly believe that the animal sector in India is poised for a giant leap through technology innovations and this status report would play a small role in highlighting the investment opportunities in this sector. This report would also be helpful in disseminating valuable information not only to industry but also for the upcoming entrepreneurs, researchers and students who are looking for business opportunities. This would also be helpful in the START UP INDIA and MAKE IN INDIA initiatives of the Indian Govt. in the Animal agriculture sector. This endeavour is a preliminary attempt towards documenting the veterinary vaccines and diagnostics in India. In this quest any omission may kindly be forgiven.

The authors would profoundly like to acknowledge the funding support of the Dept. of Biotechnology, Government of India; TANUVAS for providing all the facilities to implement this effort and M/s. Sathguru Management Consultants Private Limited, Hyderabad for their consultancy. Further the contribution of the livestock industry personnel in sharing information about the sector is also acknowledged along with all other researchers, staff and faculty of TANUVAS who have contributed towards this exercise. A special thanks for the contributions of Dr. M. Raman, Dr. B. Mohanasubramanian, P. Monisha and Manish Batham.

G. Dhinakar Raj

S.R. Rao

S. Thilagar

Contents

① Veterinary Biologicals Market

1.1 Introduction

1.1.1 Market Overview

Livestock, Poultry and Companion animals form the major animal health care markets while pigs and equines form the minor segment of the market in India. Access to high quality protein is essential to feed the growing human population and hence the need for increased and efficient livestock and poultry productivity. More emphasis and awareness of disease management is generating growth in these major markets for preventing and curative services. On the other hand, companion animal segment is witnessing improvements as a result of growing human-animal bond and thereby focusing on protecting human health by prevention of disease pathogens from animals. Livestock and poultry health sector grow as a result of adherence to food safety, disease prevention and productivity improvement principles while companion animal health sectors grows due to affordability and emotional bonding with the owner.

The global animal healthcare market is $23.9 billion today and witnesses a growth of more than 4 per cent annually [International Federation of Animal Health (IFAH)]. Market research reports predict the global animal healthcare market to exceed $ 42 billion by the end of 2019 globally, with a projected CAGR of the global animal healthcare market at 7.1 per cent between 2014 and 2019. This market comprises of three segments - pharmaceuticals, feed additives and biologicals with a global share of 62 per cent, 12 per cent and 26 per cent respectively [IFAH]. The Indian share is shown in Figure 1.1. Pharmaceuticals mainly include endoparasiticides, ectoparasiticides, antibiotics, anti-inflammatory and medicines for reproductive problems. Feed additives can be further classified into nutritional

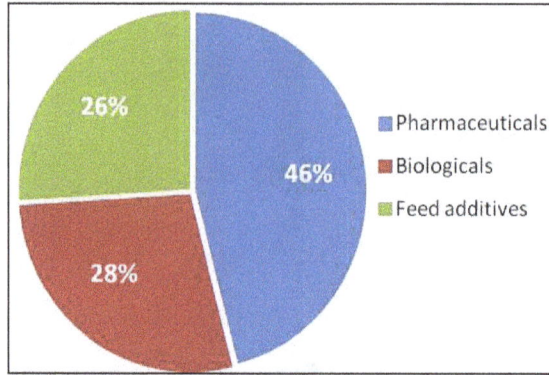

Figure 1.1: Categorization of Indian Animal Gealthcare Market by Product.

and medicinal feed additives. Nutritional feed additives comprise of vitamins, minerals and amino acids for optimal growth and production of the animals. Medicinal feed additives comprise enzymes, hormones, immune-modulators, eubiotics and feed acidifiers for specific diseases and wellbeing of animals. Globally, animal biological constitute around 26 per cent with an annual growth rate of 7 per cent of the overall animal health care market and in India this segment contributes to 28 per cent with an annual growth rate higher than 10 per cent.

Livestock comprises of cattle (cows and buffaloes), poultry comprises of layer and broilers and companion animals mainly comprises of dogs and cats. The respective animal segments are different and have unique industry operations that are characteristics of each sector. This report primarily focuses on the vaccine and diagnostic industry of the above mentioned animal sections highlighting animal population, overall demand/supply of vaccines, import-export/domestic production capability and key industry participants of the veterinary vaccine industry from manufacturers to end-consumers thereby, covering the entire value chain.

The overall animal population in India is 1,493,000 million (Table 1.1) India possesses one of the largest livestock wealth in the world with a population of close to 500 million (source: 19th Livestock census). The livestock population is scattered throughout the country with few density pockets in Uttar Pradesh, Andhra Pradesh for bovines and North eastern states for small ruminants. Majority of the livestock is owned by small and marginal farmers representing a scattered and unstructured industry.

Table 1.1: Animal Population in India

Species	Numbers (In millions)
Cattle (cows and buffaloes)	299.6
Small ruminants (sheep, goat and pigs)	200.0
Companion Animals (Dogs)	28.8
Poultry	968.0
Others	12.0
Total	**1,493.0**

On the contrary, poultry sector is a highly consolidated industry (close to 70 per cent) with majority stake controlled by few big players that have a backward and forward integration in the value chain thereby, controlling the entire industry. Livestock and Poultry have a larger share globally, with India ranking number one in livestock productivity and sixth in poultry meat production (Source: FAOSTAT-2011). In India, the public animal health care infrastructure currently available is about 10094 veterinary hospitals/polyclinics and 21269 veterinary dispensaries and 970 Animal Disease Diagnostic Laboratories (ADDL) to cater to the health and wellbeing of the animals and to ensure higher productivity and better health.

Despite India having a large population with 20 per cent of world's cattle and 50 per cent of world's buffalo population and being largest milk and 3rd largest cattle meat producer, the Indian animal healthcare combined market for all nonhuman species is 50 times smaller than the global animal healthcare market. The Indian animal health market contributes 2.2 per cent to the total global market. The reason for a smaller market contribution has been lack of adoption of innovative technologies used for prevention and cure of diseases, lack of awareness among farm owners amongst other reasons. This scenario is slowly changing with emphasis

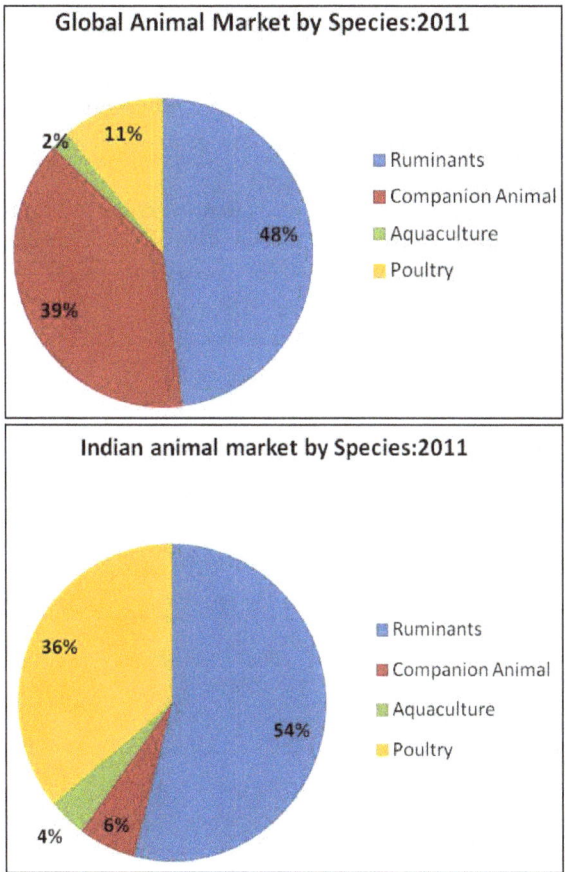

Global Animal Market by Species:2011

Ruminants 48%
Companion Animal 39%
Aquaculture 2%
Poultry 11%

Indian animal market by Species:2011

Ruminants 54%
Companion Animal 6%
Aquaculture 4%
Poultry 36%

Figure 1.2: Comparison of Global vs Indian Animal Healthcare Market by Value.

on preventive medicine and adoption of vaccination and therapeutics to enhance overall health of animals, further increasing their productivity.

The Indian animal healthcare market primarily comprises for livestock (cattle and small ruminants) closely followed by poultry industry as depicted in Figure 1.2. Companion animals make a small portion of the industry today but are the fastest growing segments registering a growth of about 20 per cent. With growing emphasis on animal health and with preventative medicine playing a major role, the Indian livestock industry is growing at a tremendous rate. The vaccination programs for livestock is mainly driven in the country today are dominated by public procurement run by the central and state governments. With the introduction of national disease control programs, a paradigm shift is seen in the industry from public institution vaccine manufacturing to entry of private players in recent years to fulfil the demand supply gap. The poultry industry, on the other hand is a highly consolidated oligopolistic industry with a few players controlling the entire industry. Other companies have made a mark in this sector with their product development capabilities and specialty vaccine portfolios. This unorganized poultry segment in the industry which contributes about 30 per cent, is mainly driven by government aided vaccination outreach programs, but is evolving further with some private companies reaching out to this untouched segment to explore further growth opportunities.

In recent years, companion animal industry has seen tremendous growth in pharmaceuticals and food segments. Vaccine and diagnostic industry has seen

Table 1.2: Current Players in the Market - Vaccine Manufacturers

Sl.No.	Organization	Vaccine Sectors
1.	Biovet Pvt. Ltd.	Livestock
2.	Biomed	Livestock, Poultry and Companion Animals
3.	Boehringer Ingelheim	Poultry and Equine
4.	Brilliant Bio Pharm Pvt. Ltd.	Livestock and Companion Animals
5.	Globion India Pvt. Ltd.	Poultry
6.	Hester Biosciences Ltd.	Poultry and Small ruminants
7.	Indian Immunologicals Pvt. Ltd	Livestock and Companion Animals
8.	Indovax Private Ltd.	Livestock and Poultry
9.	Intervet Pvt. Ltd. (Merck Animal Health)	Livestock, Poultry and Companion Animals
10.	Merial Animal Health (A Sanofi Company)	Small ruminants, Poultry and Companion Animals
11.	Ventri Biologicals (Venkateshwara Hatcheries Group)	Poultry
12.	Virbac Animal Health India Pvt. Ltd.	Companion Animals
13.	Zoetis India Ltd. (Pfizer Animal Health)	Poultry and Companion Animals
14.	Zydus Animal Health	Poultry

tremendous growth as well owing to increased urbanization in the country. With pet-owners willingness to pay and increasing pet population, the companion animal sector is one of the fastest registered growing segment in the coming decade.

A brief introduction of major players in the Indian veterinary vaccine is mentioned in the Table 1.2. The overall animal health biological market is fragmented with the top players controlling by far the majority of the market share. The market is highly volatile with considerable number of mergers, acquisitions and joint ventures taking place over the years and existing competition from smaller players is expected to reduce owing to increased integration and consolidation activities taking place.

Animal health industry has huge market worth $ 23.9 billion in world. It is growing by nominal growth of + 4 per cent. But market demand is increasing very fast because human rely on animals for food. The market of animal health can be differentiated as given in Figure 1.3. There are many companies in animal health market but demand is still growing because of different animal diseases. Some key players of animal health market are given in Table 1.3.

1.2 Indian Status

The Indian Animal Health Industry has played a vital role in safeguarding the animal husbandry interests of the nation. The Indian animal healthcare market is estimated to be around 42000 million INR (2014) and is projected to be around 60000 million by 2018. The species share in AH market is 50 per cent for livestock,

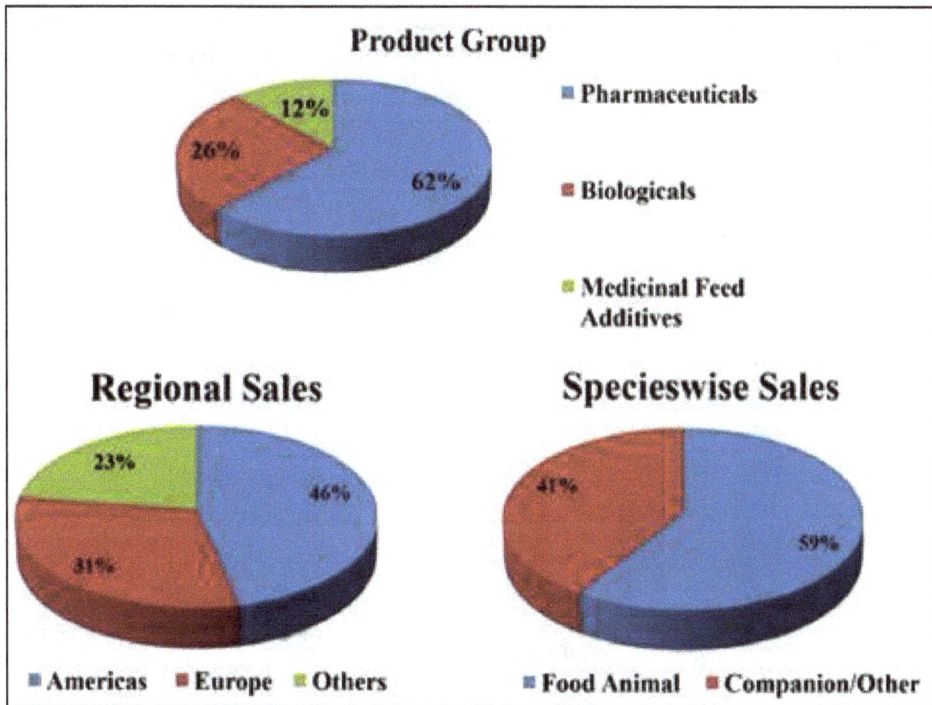

Figure 1.3: World Market of Animal Health.
Source: Global market review 2011.

40 per cent for poultry, 5 per cent for companion animals and rest 5 per cent for other remaining animals (*infah. org website*). India has 56.7 per cent of world's buffaloes, 12.5 per cent cattle, 20.4 per cent small ruminants, 2.4 per cent camel, 1.4 per cent equine, 1.5 per cent pigs and 3.1 per cent poultry (*FAOSTAT. www.fao.org*)

Table 1.3: Key Players in Animal Health Market Worldwide

Company	Revenue from Animal Health ($ Bn)
Pfizer	3.575
Merck	2.900
Sanofi-Aventis	2.635
Bayer Healthcare	0.800
Virbac	0.781
Novartis	0.500
Boehringer Ingelheim	0.354
Heska Corporation	0.065

In India the distribution of livestock is highly fragmented among the millions of rural holdings. Indian livestock production system operates on low input and output basis. Vaccines and diagnostics are two sides of same coin - Immunoprophylaxis. There is a need for expanding the range of available veterinary vaccines and also increasing their efficacy with reduced side effects. In veterinary diagnostics only a few user- friendly and cheap diagnostic kits for field use are available. The domestic animal health industry is about $ 275 million (1400 crores) as against domestic pharmaceutical market of $ 5 million *i.e.* 4.5 per cent of the market. Public sectors mainly consist of Govt. institutes with most of the states having one veterinary biological institute manufacturing vaccines for animals. The animal biological market is growing at the rate of 15 per cent against animal healthcare market of seven per cent. Animal wealth in India has increased manifold and animal husbandry practices have

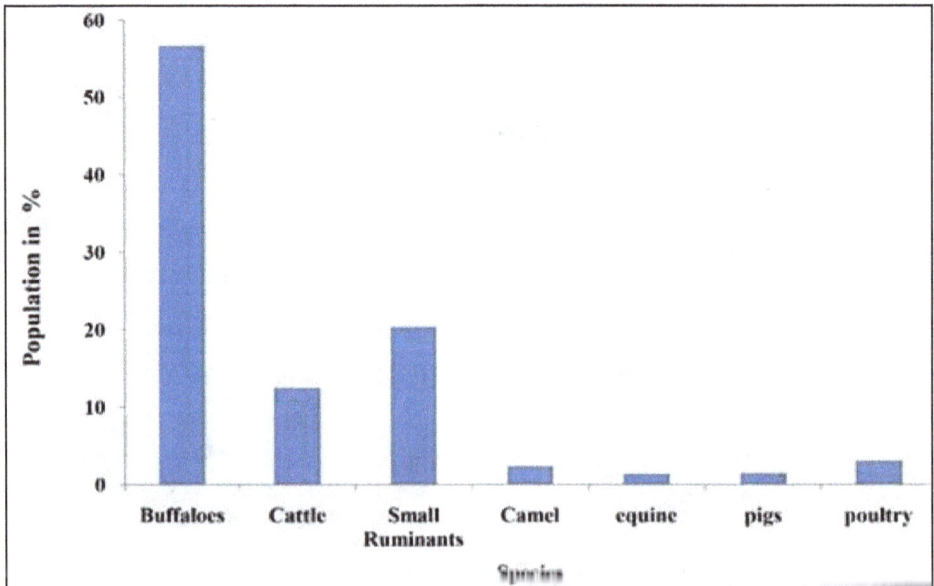

Figure 1.4: Indian Animal Population in Comparison to World Population.

Table 1.4: Animal Population in different States of India

Sl.No.	State	Bovine	Caprine/Ovine	Canine	Porcine	Poultry
1.	Andhra Pradesh	20218732	35466804	788527	394362	161333929
2.	Rajasthan	26300557	30745641	569575	237674	8024424
3.	Uttar Pradesh	50182401	16939268	766728	1334392	18667832
4.	Karnataka	12986989	14379908	1275122	304798	53442030
5.	Tamil Nadu	9594473	12930021	1547238	183983	117348894
6.	West Bengal	17112707	12582065	295714	648111	52837576
7.	Bihar	19798756	12385987	145687	649713	12748052
8.	Maharashtra	21078599	11015688	1265697	325756	77794571
9.	Madhya Pradesh	27790355	8322889	433367	175253	11904716
10.	Odisha	12347578	8094216	220405	280316	19890538
11.	Jharkhand	9916025	7164374	194909	962367	13559528
12.	Assam	10742869	6687260	527521	1636022	27216169
13.	Gujarat	20369527	6666722	253312	4279	15005751
14.	Jammu and Kashmir	3591865	5407385	145100	2421	8273709
15.	Chhattisgarh	11205449	3393530	263563	439059	23102158
16.	Himachal Pradesh	2869114	1924362	175008	5033	1104476
17.	Uttarakhand	2993890	1736169	221227	19907	4641937
18.	Kerala	1430896	1247523	923359	55782	24281928
19.	Haryana	7893428	731733	178683	126945	42821348
20.	Tripura	959600	614032	51512	362534	4272733
21.	Meghalaya	918059	493166	240638	543381	3400032
22.	Punjab	7587448	455806	470558	32221	16794076
23.	Arunachal Pradesh	732789	319087	114310	356345	2244231
24.	Sikkim	145206	115998	23314	29907	451966
25.	Nagaland	302565	103188	113021	503688	2178470
26.	Manipur	340343	76621	161818	277215	2499516
27.	Andaman and Nicobar Islands	53488	65327	27969	35921	1165363
28.	Puducherry	62005	56551	23585	1010	208721
29.	Lakshadweep	3099	46497	0	0	164541
30.	Delhi	248575	31402	150453	76346	43831
31.	Mizoram	43034	22856	39778	245238	1271353
32.	Goa	89278	12982	52323	43567	292028
33.	Dadra and Nagar Haveli	45932	4297	2109	0	85972
34.	Daman and Diu	2526	2056	503	14	28202
35.	Chandigarh	22996	871	9984	135	108719

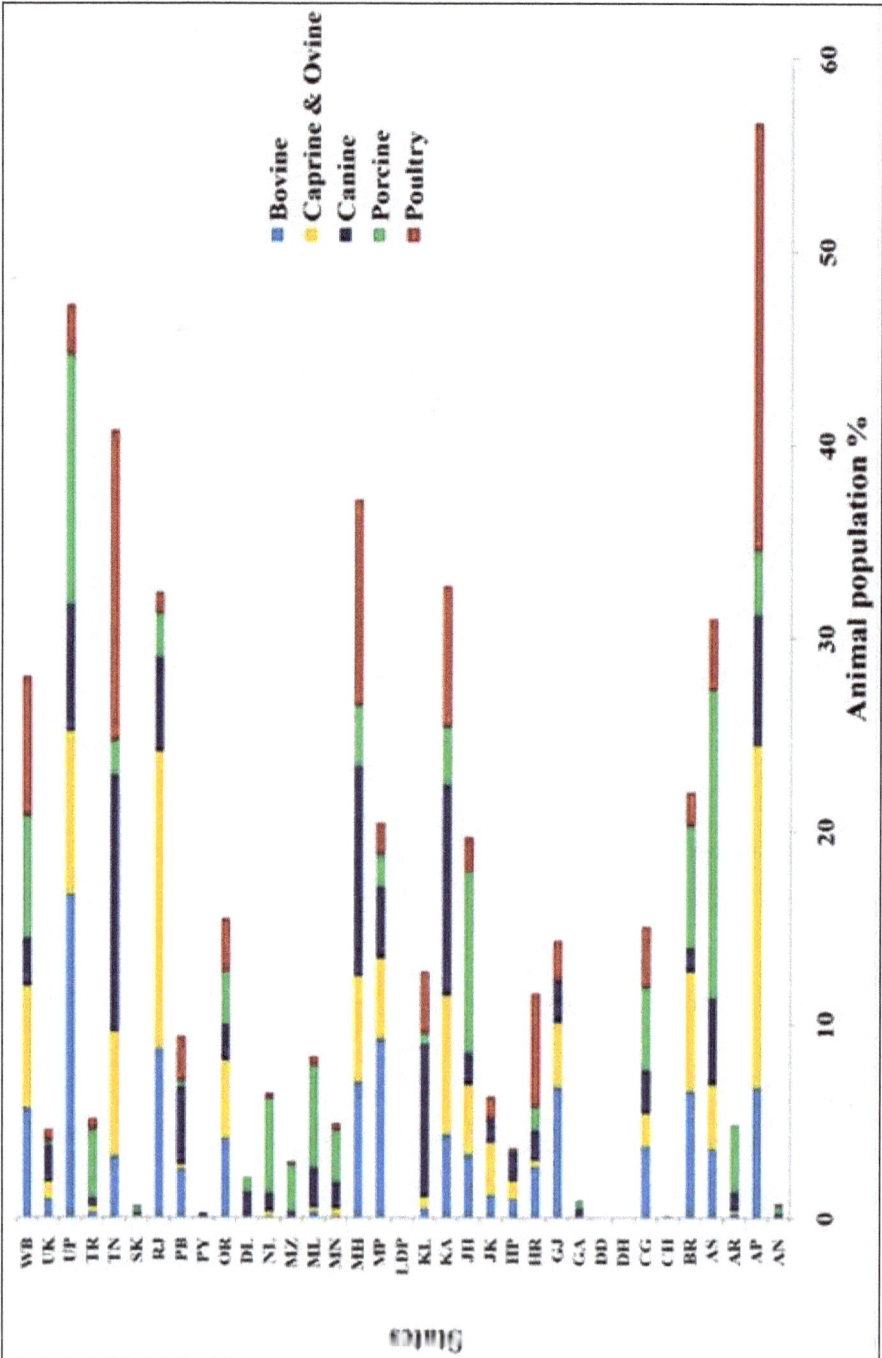

Figure 1.5: State-wise Share of Animal Population in India (in per cent).

changed following the introduction of newer technologies mostly for crossbreeding and up gradation of native breeds. In Table 1.4 and Figure 1.5 the population and per cent share of animals are given below.

India has a huge population of animal wealth. Based on figures available at the Department of Animal Husbandry, Dairying and Fisheries (*www.dahd.nic.in*), the species-wise population of different States of India was depicted in Figure 1.5. Undivided Andhra Pradesh has highest population of poultry (22.12 per cent) and Caprine and Ovine (17.71 per cent); Porcine was highest in Assam (15.89 per cent), Canine in Tamil Nadu (13.25 per cent) and Bovine in Uttar Pradesh (16.72 per cent). Lakshadweep has no population of canine and porcine. The population of poultry and bovine was reported lowest in Daman and Diu.

International Animal Health Companies (Not per ranking)

☆ Zoetis

☆ MSD Animal Health

☆ Merial

☆ Elanco

☆ Bayer Animal Health

☆ Boehringer Ingelheim Vetmedica

☆ Novartis Animal Health

☆ Ceva Santé Animale

☆ Virbac

☆ Vétoquinol

Leading Indian Animal Health Companies (Not per ranking)

☆ Indian Immunologicals

☆ Sarabhai Zydus

☆ Venkys India

☆ Intas Animal Health

☆ Alembic Animal Health

☆ Vetkind

☆ Sequent Scientific

☆ Cadila Animal Health

Common Veterinary Diseases Prevalent in India

☆ Foot and Mouth disease

☆ Black Quarter

☆ Newcastle disease

☆ Avian influenza

☆ Classical swine fever

☆ Infectious bursal disease

☆ Sheep Pox/Goat Pox

☆ Peste des petits ruminants

☆ Bluetongue

☆ Brucellosis

☆ Haemorrhagic Septicemia *etc.*

Critical Analysis of Landscape

2.1 Competitive Landscape of Animal Health Industry

2.1.1 Livestock Sector

Within livestock, this report primarily focuses on cattle and buffalo since it is the most economically important segment within livestock.

a. Market driven by public procurement and delivery by public extension to end users that largely comprise of small farms with limited capability and willingness to pay for vaccines

Majority of cattle in the country are owned by small and marginal farmers and the industry is very fragmented. The co-operative model popular in many states has supported improved market access over the years for the small and marginal farmers. Vaccination and veterinary care in this segment is largely driven by public sector extensions the marginal farm owners have negligent capability or willingness to pay for vaccination. There is also low levels of education and low appreciation of benefits of preventive care. Our interaction with some of the farmers has indicated that although the appreciation for vaccination, diagnostics and preventive as well as timely care is improving, majority of the segment still continues to have no willingness to pay for vaccines.

The same is true of other livestock animals such as sheep and goat *etc*. Hence, the livestock vaccine segment is categorized by low capability to pay by farm owners and dependence on public procurement systems. These factors also consequently result in low pricing and margins per product and given the high capex investment for live vaccines, the commercial attractiveness has historically been a deterrent to new entrants in this segment. Other than public procurement, there is no real and existing private market for livestock vaccines in this industry although the landscape might change in mid-term to long-term with international dairies investing in the Indian market and driving new and superior management practices. Today, Indian Veterinary Research Institute (IVRI) is major source of livestock vaccine production technology and as a result no product development competitive advantage exists with companies in this sector. There is no barrier to entry based on new vaccine technology and hence, it is a volume driven government procurement market with high economies of scale.

b. FMD has been the largest vaccine opportunity

The National FMD program is a government run program in the country today and is the largest commercial opportunity within livestock vaccines. The entire procurement is publicly driven with buying power in the hands of Government of India (GoI). The private companies work towards getting government tenders to fulfill the demand requirement. The FMD vaccine production is currently dominated by Indian Immunological Ltd. (IIL) and Brilliant Biopharma. Both the companies together fulfill the current demand in the country and produce about 350 million doses of the current capacity in the country of about 450 million doses. With IIL and Brilliant BioPharma announcing expansion of capacity to 860 million and 100 million doses respectively, the country's projected near term requirements should be met by the current players itself. With no significant future unmet demand in the domestic market, new entrants are either not considering FMD within cattle vaccines or are exploring export potential. For instance, Hester has set up a manufacturing plant in Kathmandu, Nepal with a focus on export of vaccines and Zoetis is focusing on producing specialty vaccines for livestock such as IBR, Brucellosis *etc.* that fill in the gap currently present in the cattle vaccine portfolio not covered in the National programs. The overall cattle vaccine market will expand in the near term with the implementation of new national programs for PPR, HS, BQ, Brucellosis *etc.* and the dominance of FMD will reduce. In addition to implementation of new national control programs, we understand that the several Government-owned facilities that produced these vaccines are facing constraints to convert to cGMP standards and this could trigger opportunities for private players to step in.

c. Vaccination practices could potentially improve and a commercially attractive private market could emerge with corporate farms and growing international investments

The dairy industry structure in India as shown in Figure 2.1 is mainly dominated by co-operatives such as Amul and Mother-Dairy. However, in the recent years, the industry has started to experience early indicators of a paradigm shift in its operating structure with privately owned companies and integrated farms now emerging as active participants seeking aggressive growth. The private dairy farms face severe logistic challenge in milk procurement, thus fully-integrated farms with 5000 to 10000 animals, advanced management practices and niche value added products are becoming more and more common.

With an increased demand of dairy products globally and India's immense strength in large cattle population, the dairy sector is driving investments from

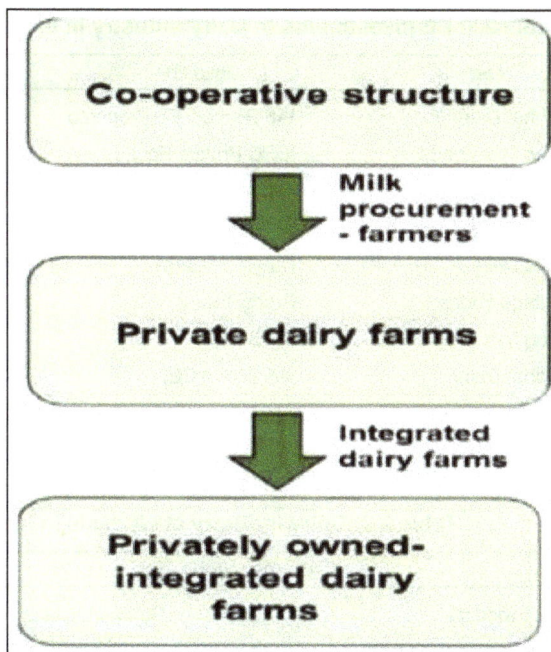

Figure 2.1: Dairy Industry Structure in India.

international firms to drive growth in long-term. The industry has not only witnessed M&A/JV's from international players but also investments from large Indian companies such as ITC foraying into dairy and juice businesses, Mahindra group consolidating all its agriculture business units into single entity to diversify its product portfolio *etc*. The backward integration with co-operatives and acquisition of private dairy farms could lead to the corporatized segment of the dairy sector emerging as a significant part of the industry in the medium term horizon. The Tables 2.1 and 2.2 summarize the investments in the last five years by various PE's and different acquisition deals by national and international dairy firms in India. This could potentially change the structure of livestock industry with private players appreciating commercial benefit of vaccination practices and driving demand for vaccines and livestock health products through direct procurement rather than through government aided programs.

2.2 Poultry Sector

The organized sector of Indian Poultry contributes nearly 70 per cent of the total output and unorganized backyard poultry in semi-urban and rural areas contributes the remaining 30 per cent. This transformation has involved sizeable investments in breeding, hatching, rearing and processing. The Indian Poultry Industry has grown largely due to private sector initiative, minimal government intervention, technical collaboration with international firms and entrepreneurial activity of small and medium farmers, and supported by considerable indigenous poultry genetics

Table 2.1: PE Investments in Dairy industry in India

Year	Target	Investor	Deal Size ($ million)
2013	Prabhat Dairy	IAF (Rabo PE), Proparco	22
2013	Parag Milk Foods	IDFC Private Equity	17
2013	Milk Mantra Dairy	Aavishkar India	1
2012	Neo Milk products	Ambit Pragma	4
2012	Dodla Dairy	Cargill Ventures	21
2012	Heritage Foods	Premji Invest	4
2012	Parag Milk Foods	IDFC PE	29
2012	Prabhat Dairy	IAF (Rabo PE)	25
2011	Milk Mantra Dairy	Aavishkar Venture	5
2010	Tirumala Milk	Carlyle Asia Growth Capital	22

Table 2.2: Dairy industry M&A deals in India

Year	Target	Stake (per cent)	Investor	Deal Size
2014	Tirumala Milk Products	100	Groupe Lactalis	275
2013	Varshney Bandhu Foods Pvt. Ltd	100	Kwality Ltd	NA
2013	Jyothi Dairy	100	Hatsun Agro Product Ltd	11
2013	Indocon Agro and Allied Activities	26	Nestle India Ltd	NA
2009	Britannia- Fonterra	49	Britannia Industries	NA

Source: VC Circle, Deal Tracker (2012-2014).

capabilities, and support from the complementary veterinary health, poultry feed, poultry equipment and poultry processing sectors.

a. Highly controlled, oligopolistic industry with dominance by two private players

The industry is oligopolistic in nature and controlled by two big players Venkateswara Group and Suguna Poultry Farms Ltd. with a large market presence. The companies have a diverse range of product and service offerings *i.e.* from chickens to eggs, farm equipment, feed and vaccine production. With their existing diversification strategy, the two companies are forward as well as backward integrated and control the entire market. Other companies that have made their presence in the poultry vaccine industry are Hester, Indovax, Intervet *etc.* These companies fill in the product portfolio gap by manufacturing specialty vaccines and focus on strategies to build in-roads into the fragmented backyard poultry. Further, a need to retain product development capability with specialized vaccines product portfolio is essential to capture their respective market shares and continued presence in this oligopolistic industry. Possibilities of additional companies entering this sector could be limited due to the consolidated nature of the industry and a strong hold of existing companies in this segment. However, these companies depend heavily on superior technologies from across the globe.

b. Active collaboration/M&A landscape: Access to technologies for Indian companies and access to market for MNC's

In the long run, the poultry industry may observe a further consolidation of the major players in the sector with new product launches, agreements, partnerships, collaborations, along with joint ventures being the most preferred strategy. The industry giants could be seen adopting these strategies to enhance their product offerings, increase their market shares and meet customer need and to consolidate their market presence. For example, international firm Merial acquired the animal healthcare company Dosch Pharmaceuticals to enter the Indian market with Merial's global portfolio of vaccine products. This acquisition gave Merial an entry to growing Indian animal health market. Poultry industry is a technology driven sector with companies having access to new technologies, gaining competitive advantage in the market. Due to this reason, companies have ventured into joint collaborations to have competitive advantage over their counterparts. For example, Lohmann Health entered into a joint venture with Globion Pvt. Ltd., Sugana's vaccine arm to expand their market in India while Suguna benefited from access to international technology.

c. Highly concentrated geographic industry pockets evolving further

The poultry industry is highly concentrated in India with few pockets specialized for broiler meat and eggs within productive states. The industry witnesses high concentration in Tamil Nadu (Namakkal for egg production and Paladam for broiler meat), Andhra Pradesh (Hyderabad and Medak for broilers) and Maharashtra (Pune belt and Nasik). The industry is growing at a tremendous rate of 10-12 per cent annually with further expansions seen towards West Bengal, Punjab and Haryana emerging as potential leading producers of poultry products.

2.3 Companion Animals Sector

a. Market dominated by international companies and is import driven

The global companion animal vaccines market is dominated by companies such as Pfizer, Merck, Virbac and Boehringer Ingelheim. The Indian companion animal sector is well evolved in terms of availability and usage of all relevant vaccines. The multinational companies import their vaccine product portfolio into India. The strategy which these companies use is a part of a broader portfolio strategy for penetrating the Indian market.

In near future, the current market size in India may not trigger companies to set-up manufacturing plants in the country for production and the companion animal vaccine market will continue to remain an import oriented, steadily growing market with an increase in demand for products. There is potentially no barrier for an international company to enter the Indian market. However due to limited opportunity for domestic manufacturing which is a high capital investment and with spread-out and scattered distribution, this market is less commercially attractive to companies. The geographic concentration of markets is predominantly urban areas with semi-urban areas potentially growing in size as attractive markets for future expansion.

b. Care for companion animals, affordability and increasing consumer buying power driving industry

The increasing disposable incomes, nuclear families with well-established and accepted pet food industry fuel the growth of the vaccine and diagnostic market in the country. With increased disposable income, there is a willingness to spend among the users, with annual spending of INR 4000-6000 on vaccines and growing at a rate of 10-15 per cent annually [Reports from Euromonitor, 2014]. Unlike the livestock sector, the buying power vests in the hands of the end customer who has buying power to drive the market.

2.4 Vaccine Industry Growth Drivers

The factors responsible for the growth of the veterinary market in India include increasing incidence of zoonotic diseases in humans; growing prevalence of animal diseases; and increasing investments by government bodies, animal welfare associations, and leading players. The strategic decisions of manufacturers in Indian environment are expected to positively impact growth in this segment. Other factors driving the growth in this space are continuous innovations and introduction of new products in the market, increasing animal population of production animals, growing prevalence of animal diseases; increasing incidence of zoonotic disease and the vaccination practices in the country. Approximately 70 per cent of the diseases known to affect humans are zoonotic and due to the growing number of people keeping pets as companions, there has been an increased risk of infections leading to an increased usage of the animal healthcare products.

2.5 Market Demand and Consumption Led Animal Population Growth

Based on the census data from 1992-2012, the livestock (bovines, pigs, goat and sheep) in the country has been witnessing minimal population growth. Although the cattle head count has remained fairly stagnant, there has been a significant increase in productivity of milk and meat from livestock. With India being the largest milk producer and one of the top buffalo meat exporting countries, the demand for healthier livestock is bound to increase in near future, thereby further driving the vaccine industry giving farmers an incentive to carry out vaccination. There is an increase in adoption of cross-bred animals in the country that are although productive but are highly disease prone. In order to maintain their productivity and reduce disease prevalence, vaccination is very important. Thus, further adoption of cross- breeds will lead to enhanced vaccination practices in the country. Thus, an increase in consumption would act as a market growth driver in future for the livestock segment. On the other hand in poultry segment, the industry is highly consolidated in nature. There has been a tremendous increase in the bird population with industry witnessing a sustainable growth rate of 12.5 per cent (19th livestock census). With an increase in urban and semi-urban population, household income, protein rich diet adoption, the increase in poultry population can be accounted to increase in consumption of eggs and meat. Thus, volume based consumption of vaccines in poultry would drive this market in near future.

2.6 Evolving Disease Profiles in Poultry Driving Product Development Landscape and Industry Growth

Several factors including animal diseases impact livestock production and productivity leading to a great impact on food supplies, trade and commerce and human health globally. The last decade has seen a significant reduction in livestock diseases due to the result of availability and effectiveness of drugs and vaccines, as well as improvements in diagnostic technologies. On the contrary, the poultry segment at the same time has witnessed the emergence of new diseases, such as avian influenza, which have caused considerable global concern. In future, infectious diseases in poultry will remain a major concern with several factors such as travel, migratory birds, trade, climatic changes *etc.* playing a major role to promote the spread of infections to new regions. Dr. Roth, Centre for Food Security and Public Health (CSFPH), a global authority indicated that swine segment is also witnessing similar evolving disease threats. With the constant evolution and onset of emerging new diseases in animals, the animal healthcare market has to remain responsive to addressing these health challenges. Thus, vulnerability to diseases such as avian influenza, and other viral and bacterial infections will steer the demand for veterinary vaccines in India. The re-emerging pattern of disease on the other hand, would be a major growth driver compelling vaccine manufactures to invest in new vaccine product development to cater to the need of the changing disease landscape.

2.7 Vaccination Practices and Vaccination Coverage Driving Significant Growth

The nationalization of the FMD control program and the initiation of several such programs by the government have led to an increased awareness and demand of the vaccines in livestock sector. With the FMD program covering the entire nation, the demand for FMD vaccine has risen in recent years. Other national programs such as for PPR, HS, BQ, Brucellosis would be potential growth drivers for livestock vaccine sector. Furthermore, recognition of new diseases and inclusion in vaccination schedules of new prevalent diseases would result in driving a demand oriented growth followed by an increased coverage for emerging diseases in the birds. The companion animal market is the fastest growing segment in India with urban and semi-urban pet population driving the growth in this segment. With the implementation of Animal Birth Control (ABC) program nationally along with other zoonotic disease vaccination for stray dogs, the sector could potentially be a huge growth factor for companion animal vaccines.

2.8 Innovation and Product Development Landscape

With prevalence of zoonotic diseases and an increased awareness among the society, the veterinary product development in recent years has seen the emergence of research efforts in vaccines and diagnostics for many of these diseases. In livestock sector, the latest technology adoption has been of DIVA FMD vaccines that enable veterinary clinicians to easily differentiate infected animals from vaccinated animals based on their antibody response to the disease antigen. Companies like BioVet and Sanvita Biotech have shown interest in furthering research for DIVA technology enabled vaccine development. There are further research engagements from government research institutes such as TANUVAS (Blue Tongue vaccine research), Animal Research Institute in J and K (research on Foot Rot vaccine) and IVRI who work on various other economically important livestock diseases. The research in this sector is primarily government funded and according to Dr. Roth not much new disease emergence in livestock sector, is comparable to global levels of product development.

In poultry sector, some of the focused research areas have been in developing new vaccines for emerging and re-emerging diseases, improving the stability of existing vaccines, discovery of new adjuvants and recombinant vaccines for better and heightened immune response. Various veterinary vaccine manufactures are actively investing in research and development for recombinant vaccines such as for poultry diseases such as IB, IBD, ND and Reo. MSD has developed a recombinant vaccine for Marek's disease with ongoing research for such specialty products for other diseases, in its pipeline.

On the other hand, in companion animals, the market is not large enough for product development and innovation efforts. The market is dominated by international companies importing their global vaccine portfolio in the country, with no Indian company entering the market in near future. The public sector is limited to rabies vaccine research and program implementation with limited research in other areas of zoonotic diseases.

2.9 Requirement to Strengthen Surveillance Practices for Zoonotic Diseases and Emerging Threats

In a country like India, where there are numerous disease outbreaks, it is very important to have a sound surveillance mechanism for effective control of animal diseases that have economic impact on the country. Today, there is a dearth of official public surveillance data in the country. Surveillance reports are a critical element of any strategy to control diseases and form the basis for initiating disease control strategies through optimal utilization of funds, veterinary resources and manpower. The current efforts of prevention and control of livestock diseases needs to be strengthened along with efficient, easy and fast regulatory approvals to market the vaccines during disease outbreaks.

For example, there is a need to strengthen surveillance of zoonotic diseases such as for Bovine tuberculosis for which animals are potent carriers and there is no current practice to identify disease spread under existing surveillance programs. Proper documentation of their disease prevalence and recognition of endemic areas for these diseases could pave way for a better vaccination practices leading to healthier animals. In poultry, Marek's disease virulent strain which is globally considered as the most pathogenic strain is also recognized in the country today. With no data for validation of the disease prevalence in the country, indicative preventive vaccination could not be carried out as per global standards.

Certain animal segments such as camels, wild animals, horses etc. are completely neglected. They should also be included in surveillance programs for better management of cross-border disease transmission. Currently, no uniform vaccination schedules are followed for these animals. The vaccines are imported and have a limited demand. The global vaccines available are of exotic strains of the pathogens and there is a need for locally relevant domestic strains for many diseases.

2.10 Unmet Need in Product Development and Vaccination Practices

1. **Need to increase potency of FMD vaccine and current immunization practice**

With the implementation of the National FMD program in India, entire cattle population was vaccinated. In spite of national coverage, outbreaks of FMD are recorded on a regular basis. There is high need for a more potent FMD vaccine in the country and better vaccination practices. Outreach is a major issue and traceability adds a new dimension in disease management. Advanced techniques for tagging of animals such as RFID chips can be used for tracking individual animals and will be more effective. With better tagging of vaccinated animals and better coverage, outbreaks could be prevented in future.

2. **Small ruminants not covered under current vaccination programs, continue to be FMD carriers**

The small ruminants that are currently not covered under the national FMD program pose a threat in eradication of FMD in the country. These animals are active carriers of the disease and spread it to larger ruminants like cows and buffaloes. Without addressing the need of vaccination programs for small ruminants, it will be a challenge to eradicate FMD from the country. Other livestock diseases such as **sheep pox, goat pox, PPR and Bluetongue** are some of the most prevalent diseases in these animals and require the support of government bodies for their control and eradication.

Other animal segments that need attention are equines, camels, wild animals and exotic pet birds. A similar need has been observed for companion animal vaccines currently used in the country.

The animal diagnostics in the country today is mostly laboratory driven. There are government run diagnostic labs in each state in the country at a district level for livestock disease diagnosis that are fully equipped and functionally headed by the Joint Director. Further every taluk and block has basic diagnostic centers. There is currently a need for capacity expansion of these diagnostic laboratories. There exists a major requirement for diagnosis point of care testing devices in livestock for pregnancy and for detection of various diseases. The current diagnosis of livestock diseases are done in state government operated diagnostics laboratories with a turnaround time for laboratory test results being long and varied, thereby creating delays in critical decision making for veterinary practitioners as in Figure 2.2.

With the introduction of POCT devices and kits, diagnosis of commonly occurring diseases would become convenient and less time consuming. The challenge would be to drive adoption of POCT diagnosis in livestock segment.

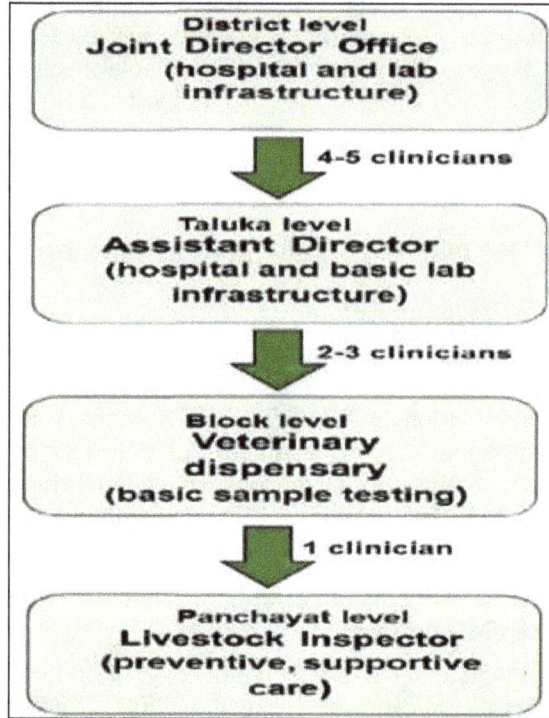

Figure 2.2: Unmet Need in Animal Diagnostics.

Contrary to companion animals, livestock is a scattered market where owners do not have a willingness to pay majorly because livestock is owned by small farmers in rural areas with low purchasing powers. Public procurement driven by government and adoption of POCT can be a major contributor of growth driver for diagnostics industry in animal health. For companion animals, there is a huge demand for the POC testing with high specificity and sensitivity of the kits with a willingness to pay by the pet owners. However the market is too small and hence the demand is not met for the animals in the country.

2.11 Constraints in the Industry

1. Regulatory Constraints and Timelines for Approvals

Serious safety issues, related to live or live-attenuated vaccines with risk of residual virulence, reversion to pathogenic wild types and likely immune suppression have resulted in stricter regulatory requirements for live or live-attenuated vaccines. Vaccine development is an extremely lengthy process in India and requires approvals from numerous agencies and committees in the government. Thus, the current regulatory framework in the country requires rigorous paper work between the central and the state government approval bodies to obtain the test licenses and manufacturing licenses. The time taken to obtain such license is extended beyond the stimulated timelines and has been deterrent for certain product launches as per the market demand. Hence, there is a need for appropriate coordination and framework for a sustainable growth of the industry. Also, on the other hand, the Indian vaccine manufacturers have the manufacturing facility with export potential which is constrained due to regulatory constraints with the import of various strains of pathogens into the country required for various vaccines.

2. Infrastructure Constraints

There exists a huge infrastructure constraint in the country today which can further be classified as follows:

a. Research Infrastructure

Research for new product development in diagnostics is mostly carried out by public institutions. There is a lack of research infrastructure in the country. On the other hand, there is lack of coordination in the triangle of researchers, farmers, extension specialists. All the stakeholders of this linage must be properly linked for impacting research creating a need for translation centers with standard practices in technology transfer. Efforts by some institutions such as Department of Biotechnology, GoI in setting up translation centers (Translational Research Platform for Veterinary Biologicals, TRPVB) at the Tamil Nadu Veterinary and Animal Sciences University (TANUVAS) would assist in fulfilling the need and lays emphasis on the need for such efforts which could strengthen product development and adoption in near future

b. Commercial Production Infrastructure

The public sector institutes governed by the State Government cater to the needs of the livestock animals of the respective State. The production capacity and details are not shared by the Government institutions and most of them are lacking cGMP facilities. Some are presently upgrading them. This has lead to shortage of a number of vaccines thereby, opening a market opportunity for the private players stepping in to fulfill the demand.

c. Supply Chain Infrastructure

The current vaccination practices are hindering continued and effective implementation of the programs. Vaccine supply chain analysis revealed an increasing maintenance costs for vaccines. Rising maintenance costs for storage of vaccines are burdening the manufacturers and distributors. The constraints in distribution of vaccines due to cold chain breakage resulting in reduced efficacy as vaccines are limiting the penetration of the market in to tier-2 and tier-3 centers.

d. Human Resource Infrastructure

There is a shortage of veterinary and para-veterinary manpower and facilities including mechanisms for diagnosis, treatment, tracking and prevention of the diseases. Adequate infrastructure for ensuring bio-security, proper quarantine systems and services to prevent the ingress of diseases across the states and national borders is not available. Lack of human resources acts as a huge constraint in the implementation of national vaccination programs, thereby making the outreach efforts difficult.

Another aspect of lack of human resource infrastructure came to our notice in the import of vaccines. The import procedure requires testing of three batches of the product at the airport which lacks required infrastructure for such undertakings with processing of only paper work.

Delays in clearance also impact the shelf life of the products thereby, reducing the efficacy of the vaccines. The import of the adjuvant, preservatives, stabilizers and other such excipients is also time consuming due to the delay in regulatory approvals and further delaying the research and development activities in the industry.

2.12 New Product Adoption Barriers

Farming is a lifestyle as it is a business, and often steeped in tradition resulting in adoption barriers of novel technologies. As most of the livestock producers are small and marginal farmers, their capacity to mobilize resources required to absorb the latest technologies developed by research institutions are limited and the adoption barrier is high in the livestock sector due to low purchasing power of the customer and their perception to prevention vs. cure needs to be evolved. The livestock sector being public sector driven with public health procurement witnesses a demand which is not strong to drive product development as the commercialization potential of the novel products developed is low due to the adoption barriers. Government procurement is not sensitive and responsive to new products with a long process to use this channel. There is currently no private procurement channel for pushing new products or any other alternate channel to reach farmers with new products. New channels are evolving with feed and small equipment companies utilizing their existing channels and offering an expanded portfolio of products.

The poultry industry is oligopolistic in nature, with product adoption governed by dominant players. The companion animal sector is a scattered market with lack of organized distribution network. Diagnostic companies like Ubio, Ggenomix have to collaborate with larger firms with the capability to reach out to clinicians in semi-urban and urban areas. Thus, lack of distribution network acts a product adoption barrier in this sector.

3

Government Initiatives and Programs

3.1 Introduction

With raising importance of animal health in India the animal husbandry practices have changed to a great extent following the introduction of newer technologies particularly for crossbreeding and up gradation of indigenous breeds. The approved outlay for the Eleventh Plan (2007-2012) for the Department Animal Husbandry, Dairying and Fisheries is Rs.8,174 crore as against the Rs.2,500 crore during the Tenth Plan (2002-2007). The Department has proposed to expand the ongoing Livestock Health and Disease Control (LH and DC) scheme including the National Control Program for major diseases like FMD, PPR and Brucellosis. By initiating major health schemes to support animal health programs, India has been striving to ensure disease-free status for various livestock diseases and to be compatible with the standards laid down by the Office International des Epizooties (OIE) - World Animal Health Organization to promote its livestock trade. As the knowledge of the epidemiology of any contagious disease is essential for initiating disease control strategies and the successful implementation of effective disease control programs, wide-ranging programs for systematic control of major cattle diseases of national importance are under implementation, covering Foot-and-mouth disease (FMD), Brucellosis, PPR *etc.* A network of 24 veterinary biological units in the public and private sector produce above 1000 million doses of vaccines/ sera for combating major disease of livestock and poultry.

3.2 Rinderpest

Rinderpest is a highly infectious viral disease (Morbilli virus infection) of cloven hoofed animals inflicting heavy mortality in bovine.

Control Program

The Rinderpest Control Program was launched in India during the year 1952 as a part of the second five year plan with an objective to eradicate Rinderpest and Contagious Bovine Pleuro Pneumonia (CBPP) by strengthening the veterinary services across the country and to obtain freedom from rinderpest and CBPP infection following the pathway prescribed by Office International des Epizooties (OIE), Paris. Since initiation, the program has been under execution adopting various strategies. The National Project for Rinderpest Eradication (NPRE) was launched with effect from May, 1992. The project was initially funded by the European Economic Community (EEC) until 1998 to support the Global Rinderpest Eradication program and later 100 per cent centrally sponsored. India has been free from clinical Rinderpest since June, 1995 and as per norms, India submitted the dossier on August, 2005 for obtaining freedom from Rinderpest. The International Committee of World Organization for Animal Health OIE recognized India as free from Rinderpest infection on 25th May, 2006.

3.3 Foot and Mouth Disease (FMD)

Foot and Mouth Disease is a highly contagious disease caused by apthovirus and affects the cloven footed animals, including cattle, sheep, goat and pigs. There are three serotypes, O, A and Asia 1 are prevalent in the country with Type "O" causing 70-80 per cent of the outbreaks followed by A and Asia1 while the fourth serotype C was last recorded in 1995 [The Application of a National Laboratory Network in India for Foot and Mouth Disease, PDFMD, OIE] and hence has been discontinued from vaccine preparation since October 2006. The incidence of FMD is higher in winter months and during pre-monsoon.

Among the countries listed by OIE, India had the highest incidence of FMD with 194 cases from January to December 2014. According to the latest research conducted by ICAR on FMD in livestock, the country is losing directly Rs 18,000 crore and indirectly Rs 30,000-35,000 crore annually. Apart from this, presence of FMD affects the export potential of the livestock industry due to the trade barrier, preventing export of livestock and their products, to the countries, which are free from this disease. According to the reports of The Project Directorate of Foot and Mouth Diseases (PDFMD), FMD is the biggest impediment to growth of livestock sector.

Control Programs

Recognizing the economic impact due to the disease, two FMD programs have been implemented in the country:

1. FMDCP u program that is completely funded by the government of India for the control of FMD nationally in Livestock.

2. Assistance to States for Control of Animal Diseases (ASCAD) Program of GOI and State Govt. implemented in Non FMD states

The FMD control program has been launched by the Government of India during the 10th year plan covering 54 districts and 30 million animals and pigs. The program has expanded to 167 districts in the 11th year plan and is currently expanded to cover over 121 districts and does not include the small ruminants (Figure 3.1). Under the 11th Five-Year Plan, the Ministry of Agriculture, Government of India has allotted Rs 1,200 crore to fight FMD. ICAR has decided to propose an economic assistance of Rs 4,000 crore for the same in the 12th Five Year Plan (2012-17) as the FMD program is expected to cover all the 640 districts and 316 million animals. ICAR has made the country self-sufficient, for the requirements of the FMD control program in the area of diagnosis, surveillance and monitoring and two institutions of ICAR, the Project Directorate on FMD at Mukteswar and the Bangalore Campus of Indian Veterinary Research Institute are working exclusively on FMD to provide all the required technical support to the DADF and the state Governments, for the implementation of the FMD Control Program (FMDCP).

Currently the vaccines available for FMD are killed virus vaccine which need to be injected twice a year in cattle as it provides protection for six months against the disease and during 2012-13, as against target of 110 million vaccinations, about 93.2 million vaccinations have been carried out up to December, 2012 [DADF, Annual report 2012-2013].

With an estimated demand of 600 million doses in the country, the current existing production of the FMD vaccine in the country is about 440 million doses

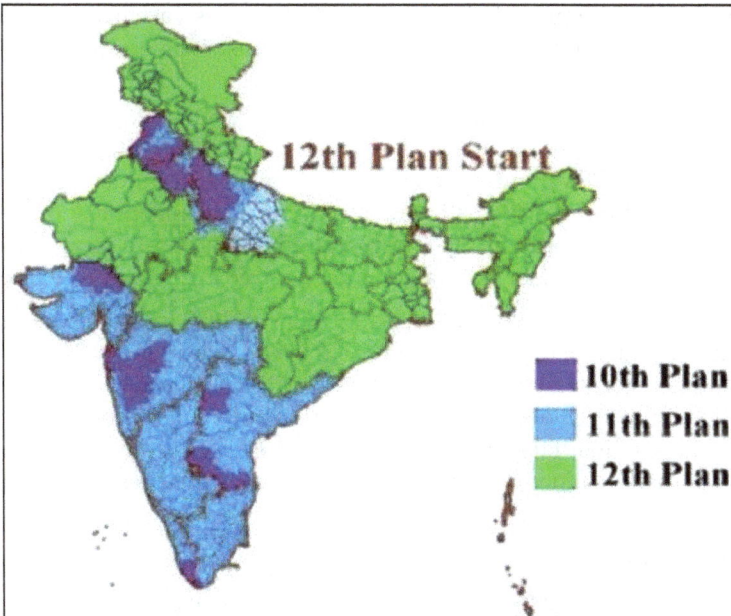

Figure 3.1: FMD Control Program Outreach.

of trivalent vaccine per annum as against the demand of 600 - 800 million with an expected to increase up to 1050 million doses in the next few years with the expansion plans of the private manufacturers as listed below in Table 3.1.

Table 3.1: FMD Vaccine Manufactures in India

Organization	Present Capacity (million doses)	Future Capacity (million doses)
Indian Immunologicals Pvt. Ltd.	250	860
IVRI	10	100
Brilliant Bio Pharma Pvt. Ltd.	100	100
Bio-Vet	40	40
Intervet	50	50
Total	450	1150

3.4 Brucellosis

Brucellosis is an economically important zoonotic disease caused by *B. abortus, B. melitensis, B. suis, B. ovis* leading to abortions and infertility in animal and has become endemic in most parts of the country. Prevention of brucellosis is of importance to reduce the abortions and to add new calves to the animal population leading to enhanced milk production.

Control Program

The National Control Program on Brucellosis has started in 2010 with 100 per cent central assistance provided to States/UTs for mass vaccination of all female calves between 6-8 months in the areas of high disease incidence.

3.5 Peste des Petits Ruminants (PPR)

Peste des Petits Ruminants (PPR) is a viral disease caused by peste des petits ruminants virus (PPRV) and characterized by high fever, mucopurulent nasal discharge, stomatitis and enteritis and diarrhea. The infection with this virus causes morbidity and mortality in sheep and goats leading to huge losses in the rural economy. PPR is widely prevalent and endemic in almost all parts of India.

According to OIE reports, the rough estimate of PPR caused economic losses is 1,800 million Indian rupees (US$39 million) every year in India. This estimate is based on information available in the literature on PPR outbreaks without laboratory confirmation. The prevalence of PPR based on the outbreaks reported is illustrated in Figure 3.2. Baseline data on the prevalence of PPR indicate that one third (33 per cent) of small ruminants in India test positive for the presence of antibodies against PPR.

Control Program

The National Control Program of PPR started in 2010 with 100 per cent control assistance involves intensive vaccination of susceptible sheep, goats and three subsequent generations. The control program for PPR would run in three phases

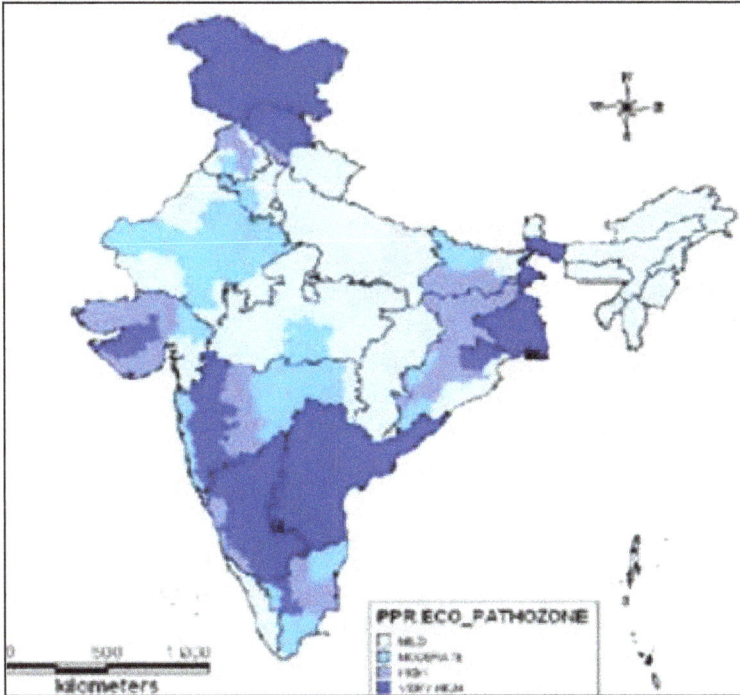

Figure 3.2: Status of PPR in India.
Source: **Project Directorate on Animal Disease Monitoring and Surveillance (PD-ADMAS), Annual Report 2011-12.**

during India's 11th (2007–12) and 12th (2012–17) 5-year plan periods. The total demand for PPR vaccine is about 200 million doses with future expectations of demand surge due to the national PPR vaccination program expansion to all states. Currently, the vaccine is manufactured by public institutions such as IAH and VB, Bengaluru; VBRI, Hyderabad *etc.* run by state governments. A few companies such as IIL, Brilliant Bio Pharma and BioVet also manufacture PPR vaccine. BioVet currently manufactures 50 million doses and plans to expand to another 50 million. A notable change in shift of PPR production from public to private sector is due to the implementation of National PPR program. Currently, Hester and MSD health plan to enter livestock vaccine manufacturing with a focus on PPR vaccine.

3.6 Hemorrhagic Septicemia (HS) and Black Quarter (BQ) Diseases

HS and BQ caused by *Pasteurella multocida* and *Clostridium chauvoei* respectively are economically important diseases of livestock and the national program for vaccination of animals have now been initiated in the country for disease control. The disease prevalence with reference to the number of outbreaks is illustrated in Figure 3.3.

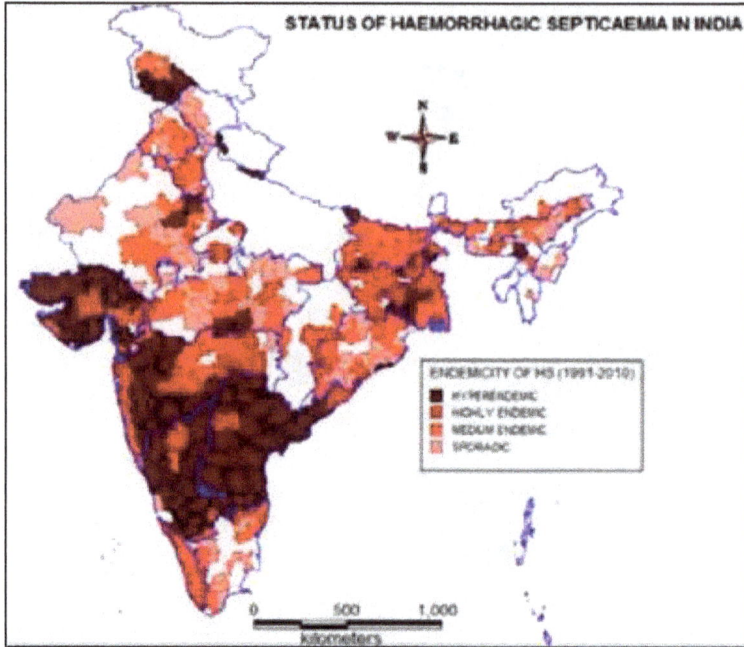

Figure 3.3: Status of HS in India.
Source: **Project Directorate on Animal Disease Monitoring and Surveillance (PD-ADMAS), Annual Report 2011-12.**

Control Programs

Currently the vaccines for these diseases are manufactured largely by the public sector institutions and there is a major opportunity for private players to step in for manufacturing these vaccines due to constraints in the production by the public institutions. At present ring vaccination is carried in villages and mandals reporting HS, BQ outbreaks followed up by annual prophylactic vaccinations for next 3-4 years or longer. The total demand for HS/BQ vaccine is close to 250 million doses. Today, the production is fulfilled by public institutions mostly, which manufacture this vaccine to fulfill demand for their respective states. For example, IVPM manufactures 120 million doses of HS/BQ vaccine to fulfill the demand in Tamil Nadu. BioVet is another manufacturer producing HS/BQ vaccine with a supply of 150 million doses to the central government procurement program.

3.7 Classical Swine Fever (CSF)

Classic Swine Fever (CSF) is an endemic disease in India with maximum outbreaks recorded in the North-Eastern States of the country, where there is a substantial pig population as depicted in Figure 3.4. Sporadic outbreaks of CSF are also reported from other parts of the country and ILRI reports have indicated that pig farmers in India incur huge losses from mortality, treatment and replacement costs - over 2 billion INR in 2012.

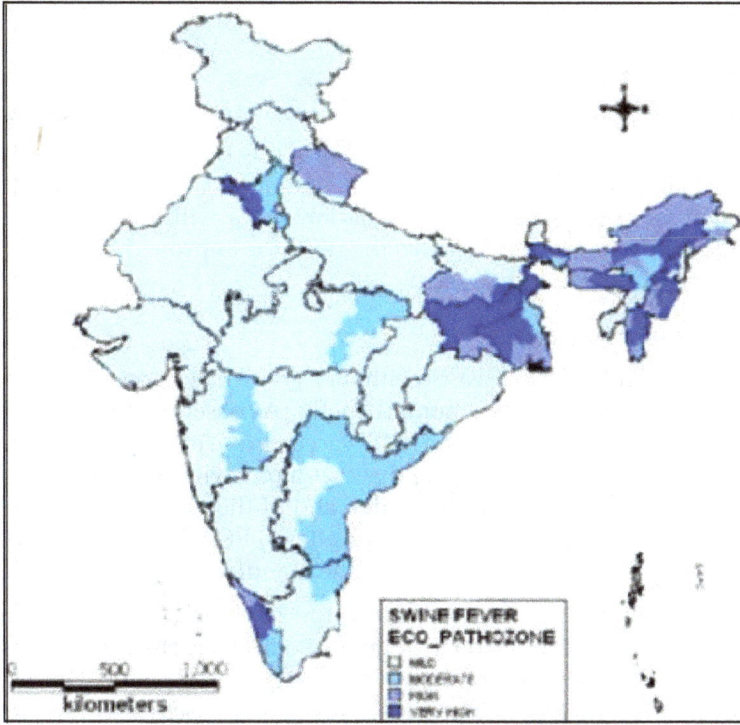

Figure 3.4: Status of CSF in India.
Source: **Project Directorate on Animal Disease Monitoring and Surveillance (PD-ADMAS), Annual Report 2011-12.**

Control Program

About 3 lakh doses by IVRI, 1 lakh doses by Institute of AH and V Biologicals, Mhow, 19,000 doses by Veterinary Biological Institute, Guwahati and the remaining by other State Biological Production Centres, particularly in the East and North-East of the Country manufacture lapinized vaccine against CSF. Attempts are being made to develop a cell-culture based vaccine for CSF which will be the only alternative to save pigs from this disease.

In order to control the classical swine fever in pigs, a new component named as Classical Swine Fever Control Program has been initiated with funds on 100 per cent central share basis are provided to the States/UTs for carrying out the vaccination of entire eligible pig population in a phased manner starting in NE states. Depending on the vaccine availability, the scope will be enlarged to cover entire country subsequently but the vaccine is not sufficient and is facing constraints its production. India requires a total of 22.26 million doses of CSF vaccine per year, with northeast India alone requiring 7.64 million doses [Classical swine fever in northeast India: Prevention and control measures, 2012, ILRI].

3.8 Drivers and Opportunities

1. Large Population

The livestock population especially the milch cattle has witnessed a growth of 6.75 per cent from the previous census. The growing demand is currently met by increased productivity of the animals which is significantly less than the threshold of productivity. An increase in the population along with the need for increase in the productivity further necessitates the need for improved health driving the vaccine industry of the livestock sector.

2. Government Programs

The burden of infectious diseases continues to be a major constraint to sustained agricultural development and economic benefits. As observed in the above section regarding the surge in demand of the FMD vaccines due to the government control programs to control and eradicate the diseases along with the initiatives taken by the private player to fill the gap in the demand of the vaccines required, similar pattern is expected with respect to the Brucellosis, PPR, CSF vaccines as per our interactions with the private livestock vaccine manufacturers.

Although most of the vaccination of the livestock is undertaken by the Government of India in their national programs, some of the emerging diseases in the country are yet to be identified by the government for their national immunization such as Bovine tuberculosis, Leptospirosis, Johne's diseases *etc.* Apart from FMD, Brucella and CSF which are well recognized and provide existing opportunities, there remain vaccine opportunities for porcine circovirus, as well as for porcine reproductive and respiratory syndrome virus, subject to government approvals recognizing the diseases for the vaccination schedules. Very few public institutes manufacture HS, BQ, CSF and Bluetongue vaccines in the country. In addition, IIL and BioVet manufacture Bluetongue vaccines. Identification of the strains prevalent in the country and recognition in the national immunization program would increase the demand for these vaccines.

These national vaccination programs have led to an increase in awareness in turn leading to an increased demand for the vaccines in the country and the emergence of additional national vaccination programs. This increase in demand would pave way for new entrants and capacity expansion of the current players in the vaccine industry. Awareness in the owners of the backyard cattle will also lead to increased use of the vaccines through improved rural penetration thereby creating an opportunity for the growth of the livestock vaccines in the country.

Department of Biotechnology, Government of India for the last two decades has been promoting basic and translational Research in universities and institutions with approximate investment of about up Rs 40 crores per year on development of vaccines and diagnostics. The projects range from individual investigator-driven competitive R&D projects, national Networks, centres and platforms.

Two important success stories are described below:

The Network Program on Brucellosis in 12 research institutes, state veterinary universities, central university *etc.* involving nearly 86 researchers is a landmark national program aimed at brucellosis control and eradication in India. There are fifteen sub-projects under DBT - Network Project on Brucellosis working on different aspects such as Epidemiology, Diagnostics, human and animal Vaccines, Brucella bacterial Repository, genomics and Bioinformatics. All the units of the network program are coordinated by a Project Monitoring Unit. The network program has completed its first phase successfully. As an outcome, a repository has been established for storing and cataloguing different Brucella species, a novel pen side diagnostic, a lateral flow assay kit, an indirect ELISA kit against Brucella species and a hand held ELISA reader have been developed.

Based on the outcome, Government of India is launching a " Brucella Free Village" involving NGOs and farmer organisations to educate the farmers in rural area, State, Central and local Animal Husbandry Departments

Translational Research Platform for Veterinary Biologicals (TRPVB)

Translational Research Platform for Veterinary Biologicals (TRPVB) is a unique partnership initiative in the naïve field of translational research between the Department of Biotechnology (DBT), GoI and Tamil Nadu Veterinary and Animal Sciences University (TANUVAS), a premiere State Veterinary University (www. trpvb.org.in)

The Vision of TRPVB is "To foster 'Productization' in the field of Veterinary Biologicals by converging the presently distant academic research, industry and pathways of regulatory compliance"

And its mission is to "Translate veterinary vaccines, diagnostics and other biologicals for field application and harness their benefit to improve animal health and productivity thereby augmenting the economic status of farmers". The mandate of TRPVB is to:

☆ Facilitate the conversion of potential leads into marketable veterinary biologicals through appropriate production and validation processes in compliance with regulatory requirements

☆ Provide regulatory compliant biotechnological services and technical assistance for industry and academia.

☆ Attaining the status of knowledge and information hub on veterinary biologicals

TRPVB has been trying to bridge the translational disconnect between academia, industry and regulation over the last 5 years. Some of their approaches include

TRPVB a Unique Amalgamation of Expertise

☆ TRPVB has made a unique attempt to bring in academia/industry and regulatory experts who can leverage and assist clients in various stages of product development

☆ Being housed in one of the leading Veterinary Universities in India it would provide the much needed academic ambience and act as a knowledge hub for information resources

TRPVB Laboratory: A State of Art Facility

TRPVB has established the following facilities

☆ A general laboratory

☆ GLP- clean room facility for animal cell culture and hybridoma production

☆ A dedicated BSL-2 laboratory for handling selected bacterial pathogens

Cleanroom Facility (Seamless Transition of Products)

Academic institutions in India including TANUVAS is focusing on the development of newer and better diagnostic and control measures against the infectious diseases of animals. Though the academic institutions of India possess adequate scientific acumen to develop the technologies, unavailability/inaccessibility of structural requirements impede them in meeting the quality standards. This impose additional burden on the manufacturing companies which acquire the technology from any academic institution. The companies need to repeat the seed development and other testing procedures at their cGMP certified facility as per the stipulated regulatory norms, and these processes often take years to complete. To fill this gap and also to facilitate seamless transfer of the technologies from the academia to industry, TRPVB-TANUVAS had created a state of art clean room facility meeting cGMP norms.

Biosafety Laboratory

TANUVAS is contributing considerably for the animal health in developing and validating vaccines and diagnostic kits, and also by providing disease monitoring and surveillance services. The BSL II facility of TRPVB can be used to handle high risk category organisms causing Tuberculosis or Brucellosis. The facility is equipped with all the necessary bio-containment needs such as Class II B2 Biosafety cabinet, double-door autoclave, unidirectional air flow, *etc.*

GLP Compliant Studies

Good laboratory practice (GLP) is a standard by which laboratory studies are designed, implemented, and reported. GLP practices provide assurance to the public and customers that the results are correct and the experiment can be reproduced exactly, at any time in the future. GLP practices of laboratory-based activities in an organization pride itself on the quality of the work it performs and improves customer confidence. In this aspect, TRPVB had conducted five GLP studies for three of its clients (M/s Kemin Industries, Inc., National dairy development board (NDDB) and Defense Research and Development Organization (DRDO)). All these studies were done as per GLP *i.e.*, starting from protocol preparation to final document preparation and archiving the study at TRPVB.

Joint/Co-development

TRPVB is engaging various industries in co-development of products and technologies. Engaging the industry during the development and validation stages of the product had created a participatory ecosystem for industries and this might enhance the industry's assertion on the product during the commercialization process. Industry is benefited by the expertise of TRPVB-TANUVAS and also gets access to the vast clinical and farm samples.

TRPVB is jointly developing PPRV vaccine, Nano-NDV and Brucella ELISA along with industrial partners.

Technology Acquisition

Intellectual properties and product leads at various stages of development are acquired by TRPVB and for facilitating commercialization. This provides a much needed hand holding for the fund constrained academic investigators with promising product leads. TRPVB can hasten the market influx of such leads through well-defined evaluation studies with regulatory compliant documentation. TRPVB had already acquired reproductive probiotics and Brucella ELISA and are performing regulatory compliant validation studies of these products.

Commercialization Strategies

To meet the mandate and bridge disconnect between academia and industry TRPVB operates on six different strategies to assist stakeholders at various stages of product development, in order to convert a research lead into commercial technology or product. In its Relay Mode, TRPVB nurtures a product from development until commercialization using its internal funding. In addition, TRPVB also develops products through external research grants. The product/process developed by an innovator is validated (paid service strategy) at TRPVB to enhance its commercialization potential. Further TRPVB also allows any innovator to develop his technology during its early stages by providing the much needed infrastructure through its technology incubator strategy. Moreover, TRPVB also contributes to the biotech industry and the society by offering various biotechnological services and by direct sale of products which are yet to be taken up by the industry to make it available to the people.

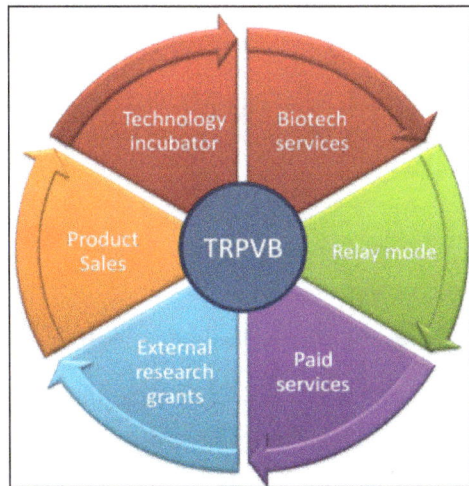

TRPVB is reinventing itself with the requirements of industry for the mandate of product development and is already making a small 'dent' in the field of Animal Sciences research commercialization !!!

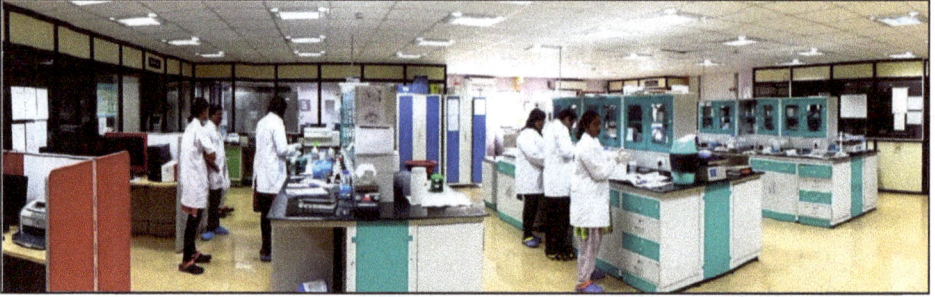

TRPVB Laboratory.

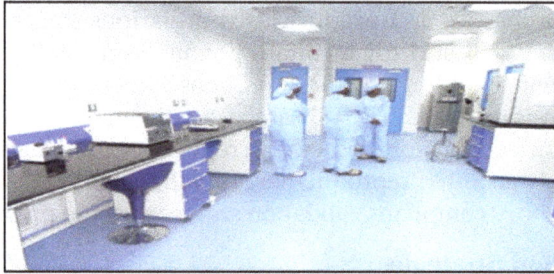

Clean Room Facility at TRPVB.

Biotechnology Industry Research Assistance Council (BIRAC) is a Government of India initiative to bridge the industry – academia interface through the following strategies

- ✰ Targeted funding for collaborative schemes
- ✰ Tech transfer
- ✰ IP management
- ✰ Hand holding schemes that create innovative competitiveness

Some of the BIRAC programmes include

- ✰ Biotechnology Ignition grant scheme
- ✰ University Innovation cluster
- ✰ Small Business Innovation research initiative
- ✰ Biotechnology Industry partnership programme
- ✰ Contract research scheme

The Technology Development Board (TDB) of the Department of Science and Technology (DST) is a statutory body, to promote development and commercialization of indigenous technology and adaptation of imported technology for wider application. The objective of TDB is commercializing of the fruits of indigenous research (http://tdb.gov.in). The main aim of TDB is to facilitate interactions between academia and industry by fostering an innovation culture and provided a platform for generation of entrepreneurs.

2. Export Potential

There exists an opportunity for the Indian vaccine manufacturers to export the vaccines produced in the country to foreign markets as most of the Asian countries have similar strains of the pathogens. As per our discussion with the management of Hester Biosciences, they have indicated an interest to explore opportunities to enter cattle vaccines and plans to set up a manufacturing plant in Nepal with a capacity of 1.5 million doses for exports. Brilliant Bio Pharma Pvt. Ltd. is currently exporting their vaccines to several Asian and African countries and is keen on exploring more such opportunities. Our conversations with Dr. Roth, Center for Food Security and Public Health (CFSPF) also indicate a potential for export to countries with similar pathogen strains for routine vaccinations and emergency backup vaccinations during outbreaks, indicating a high potential for expansion for manufacturers.

Indian vaccine manufacturers did not explore Asian, African and middle-eastern market, even though these region have similar strain prevalence. The growth of the manufacturers will depend on the exports in future. The limitation to export vaccines from India would be the limited strain accessibility in the country due to the regulatory constraints to import live strains of the pathogen not prevalent in the country for vaccine manufacturing. Hence, the vaccine manufactures need to develop strategies for growth with limited strain accessibility.

3.9 Challenges and Restraints

1. Supply Chain Constrains

In spite of the ambitious disease control programs launched by the Government of India and State Governments to directly prevent the outbreak and indirectly improve productivity, there was no significant breakthrough in improving the productivity both in the milch and meat sectors and in reaching the poor for their livelihood. There is still poor attention to animal health as no other programs other than FMD are run on a large scale and in spite of the program being run on a national level, there is no data on the number of animals vaccinated. Frequent FMD outbreaks have been reported in the country and FMD has been recognized as one of the most widely reported disease in the country [Annual report 2011-12, PDADMAS]. These outbreaks in spite of the vaccination programs could be due to several factors such as issues on manufacturing, live vaccine pathogenicity, supply chain breakage. Targeted measures to reduce the occurrence of infectious diseases and quality veterinary vaccines should be a part of the government sanctioned-programs along with vaccination campaigns being a part of the comprehensive disease control program which also require regional approach for transboundary animal diseases.

2. Low Return on Investment (ROI)

A major constraint for the vaccine manufactures in the livestock sector is low return on investment (ROI) due to public procurement of the vaccines. Public procurement and low pricing could be a deterrent in profits and large volumes could create commercial feasibility and attractiveness by compensating for low margins. Emphasis on animal health and improved vaccination practices would foster growth of the livestock vaccine industry and effective national programs with wide coverage of districts (PPR, CSF Vaccination programs) and animals (small ruminants for FMD vaccination program) could trigger volumes for industry compensating the low volumes and unduly low margins. Additionally, well-structured global pooling consortiums for procurement of cattle vaccines (that are used in public extension efforts in most countries) will help enlarge procurement volumes, create commercial attractiveness and help replicate success that Indian vaccine industry has been able to accomplish in human vaccines.

3. Lack of Awareness

Another hindrance for the growth of vaccine industry in this sector is lack of awareness and lack of willingness to pay by animal owners. The existence of small farmer markets, backyard cattle, dispersed markets, poor and high costs transportation infrastructure, limited and unreliable cold chain puts pressure on the distribution costs of the manufacturers. Though the manufacturers take utmost care of cold supply chain till the vaccines reach the end customer, the supply chain breaks due to infrastructural issues such as storage issues and lack of power back up at the lower end of the chain. These issues deter the private industry entry into the livestock manufacturing which could only emerge if the private industry gains a larger share of the dairy/beef market. However, the lack of vaccine distribution infrastructure into rural farms will be a constraint and is anticipated that the industry would need to adopt innovative models of leveraging synergistic capabilities in seed/farm implement industry similar to models explored by cattle feed industry.

3.10 Disease Diagnostic Laboratories (Central/Regional Laboratories)

In order to provide referral diagnostic services one Central and five Regional Disease Diagnostic Laboratories have been setup/strengthened by the Central Government. The Centre for Animal Disease Research and Diagnosis (CADRAD) of IVRI, Izatnagar is working as the Central Laboratory. The Regional Laboratories are located at Kolkata (Eastern), Pune (Western), Jallandhar (Northern), Bangalore (Southern) and Guwahati (North-eastern). These laboratories

☆ Provide referral services for diagnosing various animal diseases.

☆ Study the problems of emerging diseases of animals.

☆ Undertake surveillance against emerging and exotic infections threatening the country.

The networking of these laboratories with other laboratories of the State Governments, ICAR and Universities has been initiated for better coordination and efficient disease diagnosis, monitoring and reporting.

Some selected Indian institutes involved in animal health are given below.

Indian Veterinary Research Institute (IVRI): Bareilly, India

☆ Regional Campus, Bangalore

☆ Regional Station, Mukteswar

☆ Regional Station, Kolkata

☆ Regional Station, Palampur

☆ Regional Station, Pune

☆ Indian Veterinary Research Institute Srinagar: Srinagar, Jammu and Kashmir

☆ **National Institute of High Security Animal Diseases:** Anand Nagar, Bhopal, Madhya Pradesh - 462021

☆ **Tamil Nadu Veterinary Animal Sciences University:** Madhavaram Milk Colony, Chennai - 600 051, Tamil Nadu.

☆ **Sri Venkateswara Veterinary University,** Prakasam Nagar Colony, Sri Padmavathi Mahila Viswa Vidyalaya, Tirupati -517 502, Andhra Pradesh.

☆ **Karnataka Veterinary, Animal and Fisheries Sciences University,** State Highway 15, Nandinagar, Bidar, Karnataka -585401

☆ **Rajasthan University of Veterinary and Animal Sciences,** Vijay Bhawan Palace Complex, Veterinary University Road, Near Deen Dayal Upadhyay Circle, Bikaner, Rajasthan-334001

☆ **Guru Angad Dev Veterinary and Animal Sciences University (GADVASU),** Ludhiana, Punjab 141004

☆ **National Institute of Animal Biotechnology (NIAB):** Miyapur, Hyderabad, Telangana 500049

☆ **Kerala Veterinary and Animal Science University,** Pookode, Kerala 673576.

Twining

Twinning is a common notion and has been used largely to assist capacity building and networking, and to guide communities together. The OIE (World Organisation for Animal Health) has applied this idea to laboratories to improve knowledge for the most significant animal diseases and zoonoses in regions of prime concern and, has straightly support plan to revamp the global capacity for observation, prevention and diseases control along greater veterinary governance. In India **National Research Centre on Equines** (Sirsa Road, Hisar-125 001, Haryana) is candidate laboratory for OIE twinning program on Equine Piroplasmosis.

3.11 OIE Approved Laboratories in India

Highly Pathogenic Avian Influenza and Low Pathogenic Avian Influenza (poultry)

National Institute of High Security Animal Diseases (NIHSAD) Indian Council of Agricultural Research (ICAR) Anand Nagar Bhopal – 462 021 Madhya Pradesh, India Tel: +91-755 275 92 04

Fax: +91-755 275 88 42; Email: ctosh@hsadl.nic.in

White Tail Disease and West Tail Disease

Dr A. Sait Sahul Hameed

C. Abdul Hakeem College

Aquaculture Biotechnology Division, Department of Zoology

Melvisharam-632 509; Vellore Dt. Tamil Nadu, India

Tel: +91-4172 26.94.87 Fax: +91-4172 26.94.87; Email: cah_sahul@hotmail.com

4

Market Requirement for Veterinary Biologicals

4.1 Cattle Biologicals Industry

Population

The total livestock population consisting of Cattle, Buffalo, Sheep, Goat, Pig, Horses and Ponies, Mules, Donkeys, Camels, Mithun and Yak in the nation is 512.05 million numbers in 2012 (Table 4.1), with a decrease about 3.33 per cent over the previous census. The cattle and buffalo are the major components of the livestock animals followed by goat, sheep and pigs respectively as illustrated in Figure 4.1. The cattle population is not evenly distributed among its states with Uttar Pradesh, Rajasthan and Andhra Pradesh (undivided) having the highest cattle population closely followed by Maharashtra, Madhya Pradesh and West Bengal as depicted in Figure 4.2. Small ruminants are scattered in most parts of the country with higher population in Andhra Pradesh, Rajasthan and Uttar Pradesh (Figure 4.3 (a)); while swine are largely present in Assam, Arunachal Pradesh, Tripura, Nagaland and Manipur (Figure 4.3 (b)). The livestock population in India had shown a mixed trend over the years. Cattle population had substantial increase in Gujarat (15.36 per cent), Uttar Pradesh (14.01 per cent), Assam (10.77 per cent), Punjab (9.57 per cent), Bihar (8.56 per cent), Sikkim (7.96 per cent), Meghalaya (7.41 per cent) and Chhattisgarh (4.34 per cent) in the last census as shown in Figure 4.4.

Table 4.1: Livestock Population in India

Animal	2012 Census (in thousands)
Cattle	190,904
Buffalo	108,702
Yaks	77
Mithuns	298
Sheep	65,069
Goat	135,173
Horses and Ponies	625
Mules	196
Donkeys	319
Camels	400
Pigs	10,294
Total	**512,057**

Source: 19th Livestock Census, DAHD.

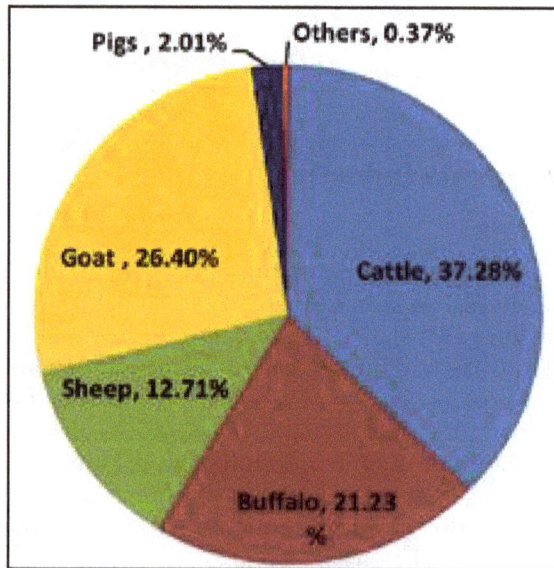

Figure 4.1: Distribution of Livestock Population in India
Source: 19th Animal Census, DADF.

4.1.1 Cattle Industry

Overview of the Industry Structure

India ranks first, accounting for 18 per cent of the world milk production and produces 132.43 million tons with an annual growth rate of 3.54 per cent. India with

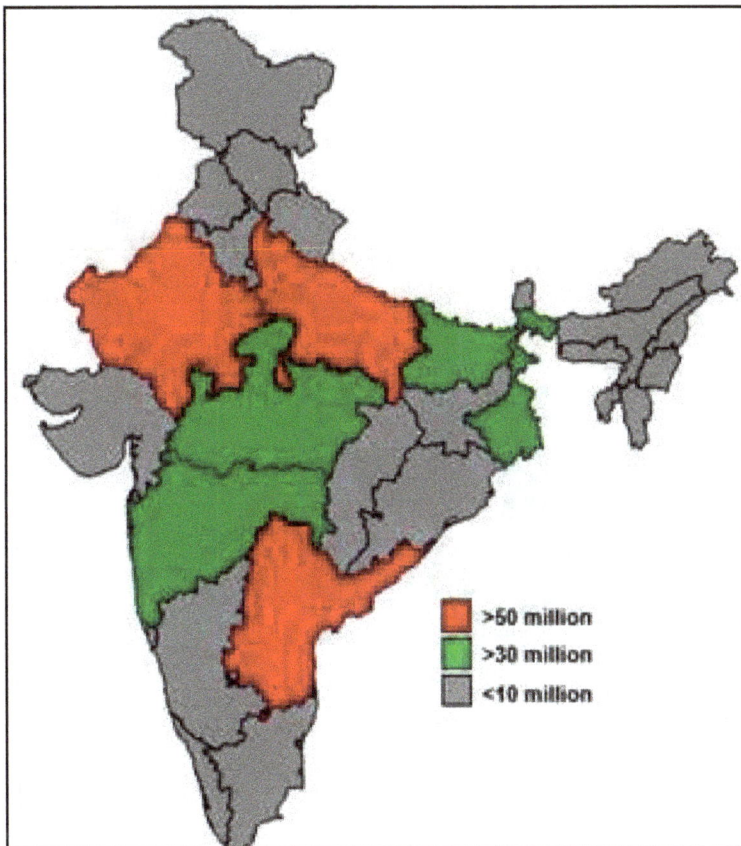

Figure 4.2: Population Distribution of Cattle in India.

its major cattle population has an emerging livestock sector and is taking steps to increase productivity. It is projected that by 2020 milk production will increase by 25 per cent respectively [PDADMAS, Vision 2030]. The per capita availability of milk is around 296 grams per day in 2012-13. Within the country, milk availability is not evenly distributed with Eastern parts of the country being a milk deficient region and the top 7 states account for 65 per cent of total milk production as illustrated in Figure 4.5 [Annual report 2012-2013, DADH].

The productivity of the Indian cattle and buffalo has been low with modest improvement over the years. The average daily milk production data at 6.52 kg for crossbreds, 2.10 kg for indigenous cattle and 4.44 kg for Buffaloes (NSSO, 2007) suggests that the productivity of these animals is far below their genetic potential and still significantly lesser than the best of global standards UK, US and Israel are at 25.6, 32.8 and 38.6 kg per day, respectively. [Balanced Feeding for Improving Livestock Productivity, FAO]. The major causes for poor productivity are due to poor nutrition/feed management, inferior farm management practices, ineffective

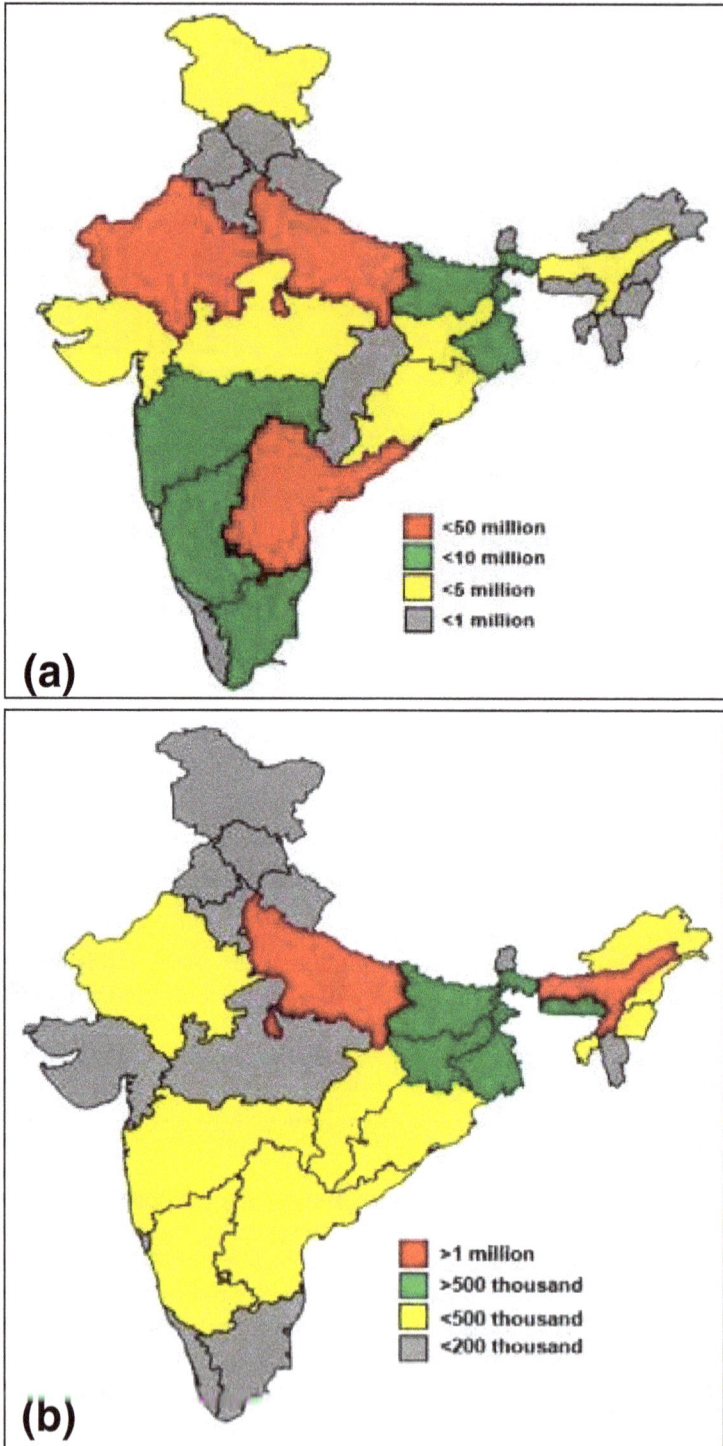

Figure 4.3: (a) Population Distribution of Small Ruminants and (b) Swine in India.

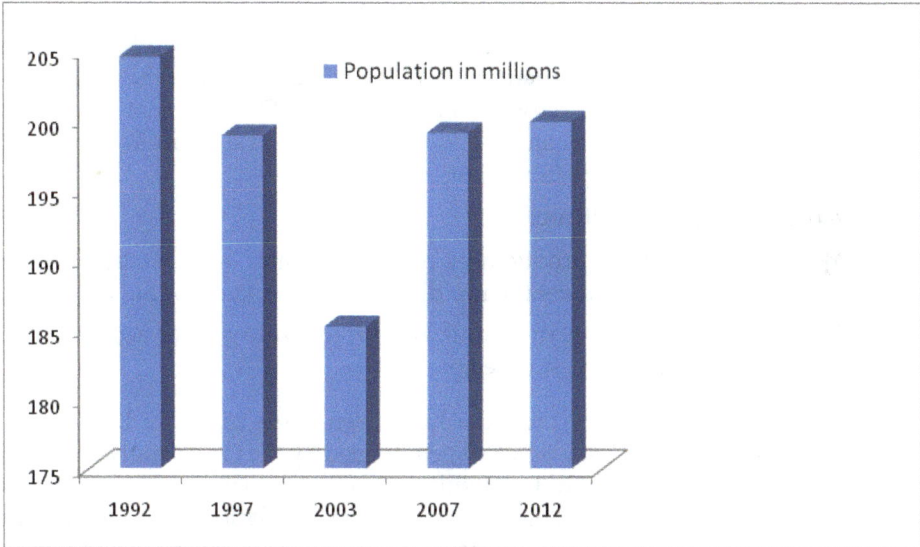

Figure 4.4: Cattle Population Census Trend.

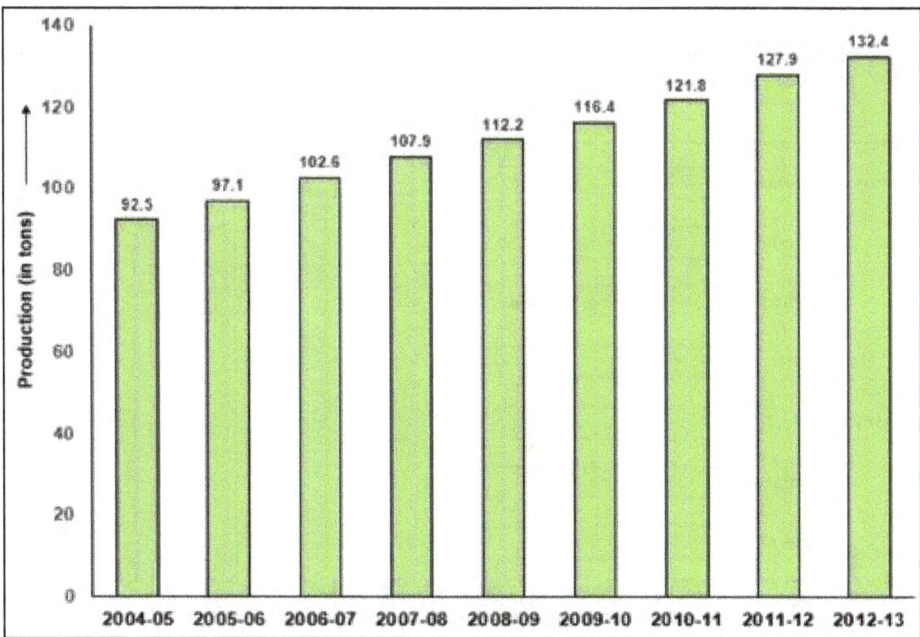

Figure 4.5: Milk Production in India (2004-2013).

veterinary and extension services in maintaining animal health and inefficient implementation of breed improvement programs.

Considering the need to meet the growing demand for milk and accelerate dairy development in the country, NDDB is implementing a National Dairy Plan

(NDP) from 2011-12 to 2018-19. NDP I will be implemented with a total investment of about Rs.2242 crore with Rs. 176 crore as Government of India share, Rs. 282 crore as share of End Implementing Agencies (EIAs) that will carry out the projects in participating states and Rs. 200 crore by National Dairy Development Board and its subsidiaries for providing technical and implementation support to the project (http://www.nddb.coop/ndpi/about/brief).

The objectives of the NDP are:

☆ To help increase in productivity of milch animals and thereby increase milk production to meet the rapidly growing demand for milk.

☆ To help in providing rural milk producers with greater access to the organised milk-processing sector.

For decades, dairy players in India have been engaged in the liquid milk processing activity only which was later spearheaded by the Co-operatives model, supported by the Government of India with top milk producing states in India as shown in Figure 4.6. With an increase of consumer preferences for value added dairy products and factors such as evolving tastes and preferences, higher affordability, *etc.*, lead to the entry of the private players taking forward the industry and the current key players are listed in Table 4.2. Besides these companies, several global dairy companies too are venturing into milk derivatives business in the country recognizing the growth potential of the sector. These companies provide veterinary

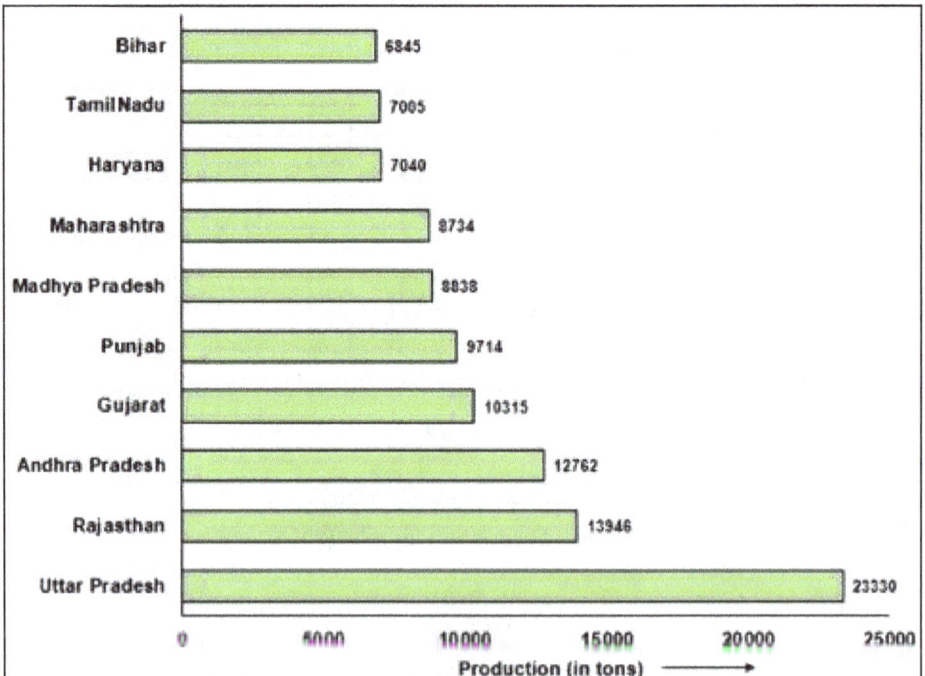

Figure 4.6: Top Ten Milk Producing States in India.

extension services and play a major role in improving the animal health and nutrition status in rural areas, to ensure high quality of milk.

Table 4.2: Key players in Indian Dairy Industry

Key Players	Brand	Revenue Turnover 2009-10 (Rs. Cr)	Revenue Turnover 2013-14 (Rs. Cr)	Vet Extension Service
GCMMF	Amul	8007	18150	Yes
Nestle India	Nestle	1641	9819	
Punjab State Coooperative	Verka	1150	1340	Yes
Hatson Agro	Anun, Komath, Cooking butter, Hatsun curd	1141	2481	Yes
Britannia Industries Ltd	Britannia	1083	6829	
Kwality	Kwality Walls	1054	4570	
Heritage Works	Heritage, Heritage Golden	900	1695	Yes
Parag Milk Food	Parag	550	1450	Yes
Modern Dairy	Modern Dairy	445	637	
Rajasthan State Cooperative	Saras	300	480	Yes
Vadilal Industries	Vadilal	189	361	
ADF Food	Ashoka	102	199	
Himalaya International	Himalaya Fresh (Paneer)	69	190	

Source: Annual reports, Business Line, Money control.

On the other hand, India's Export of Dairy products was 1,59,228.52 MT to the world for the worth of Rs.3,318.53 crores during the year 2013-14 (APEDA, Ministry of Commerce, India). India today exports to Bangladesh, Egypt Arab Republic, United Arab Emirates, Algeria, Yemen Republic and Pakistan. There is a further potential for expansion in export volume to Africa and Latin America in near future. During the last decade, dairy export has moved considerably from low value added products like milk and natural milk products to high value processed products such as cheese and yogurt. Figure 4.7 shows the percentage share in export of value added products in the last decade. These value adding products are expected to grow in near future with incoming investment from international dairy farms and P/E investors driving the industry further.

In India, buffalo, sheep, goats and pigs are major meat producing animals. Cow slaughter and beef marketing is banned in India. In 2012 the country has exported 14,49,758.64 MT of buffalo meat products to the world for the worth of Rs. 26,457.79 crores with India ranks 5th in the world in beef production, 7th in domestic consumption and 1st in exporting (Livestock and Poultry - World Market Trade, US Department of Agriculture) indicating a high growth opportunity in this industry of the livestock sector with an increasing demand and animal population. Out of the 3.643 million metric tons of beef produced in 2012, 1.963 million metric tons was consumed domestically and 1.680 million metric tons was exported. Major

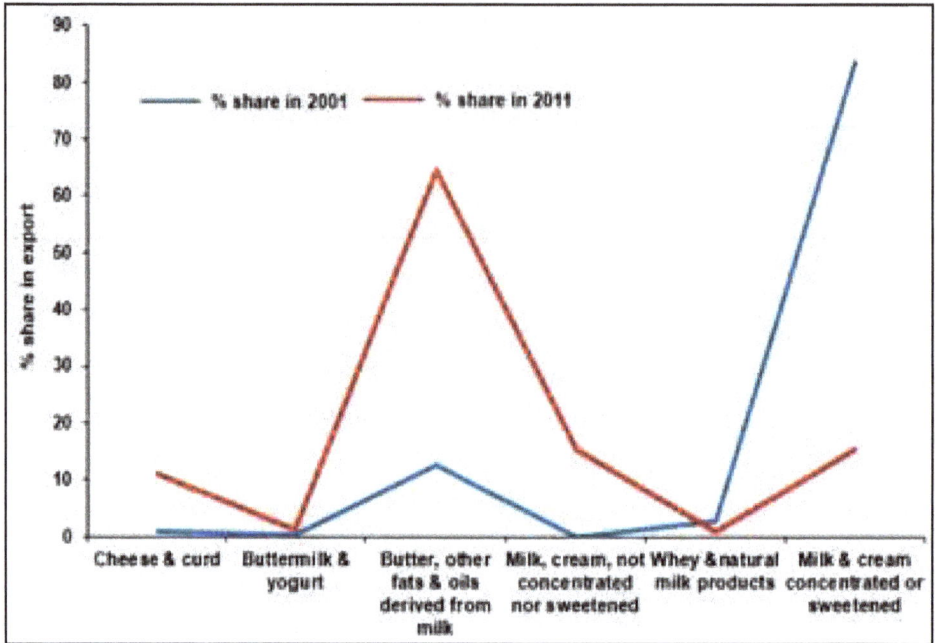

Figure 4.7: Trends in Export of Value Added Products.

beef production is from Uttar Pradesh, Andhra Pradesh, Maharashtra and Punjab [Agri exchange, APEDA].

4.1.2 Overview of Cattle Vaccine Industry

The cattle vaccine industry is the fastest emerging sector as it is primarily dependent on the Government programs with conventional manufacturing technologies. The manufacturers of the vaccines for the livestock animals are currently ramping up the capacity and predominantly the local supply due to the demand by the Government programs driving the sector. Indian Immunologicals (IIL) Pvt. Ltd and Brilliant Bio Pharma are the two key players in the livestock vaccine industry, rest being public institutions run by the state governments. IIL was setup by The National Dairy Development Board (NDDB) in 1982 for manufacturing FMD vaccine to be available for farmers at affordable prices. The technology for FMD vaccine manufacture was obtained from M/s. Wellcome Foundation Limited, United Kingdom and now manufacturers various other biologicals through their own R&D efforts. Brilliant Bio Pharma Pvt. Ltd is the second largest player in the FMD vaccine production followed by Biovet Pvt Ltd and Biomed which cater to the current demand of the FMD program followed by the other players along with the public institutions manufacturing other vaccines for large and small ruminants. Most of the vaccines manufactured by the private players (Table 4.3) are also procured and supplied by the public sector as a majority of the vaccinations are carried by the government under their national immunizations and disease control programs.

Table 4.3: Private Players in the Livestock Vaccine Sector

Sl.No.	Organization	Animal Type	Vaccine Products for Diseases
1.	Indian Immunologicals Pvt. Ltd	Livestock and Small ruminants	FMD, HS, BQ, Brucellosis, Theleriosis, PPR, Enterotoxaemia, Rabies
2.	Biovet Pvt. Ltd	Livestock	FMD, HS, BQ, PPR
3.	Biomed	Livestock	FMD, HS, BQ, Enterotoxaemia, Goat and Sheep Pox
4.	Boehringer Ingelheim	Small ruminants	Ileitis, Rabies, Porcine circovirus type-2 (PCV2), Atrophic rhinitis (PAR), Enzootic pneumonia (EP), Mycoplasma Pneumonia, PRRS virus
5.	Brilliant Bio Pharm Pvt. Ltd	Livestock	FMD, HS, BQ, Enterotoxaemia
6.	Hester Biosciences Ltd	Small ruminants	CSF, Goat Pox Vaccine, PPR, Brucella abortus
7.	Indovax Private Limited	Livestock	PPR, Brucellosis
8.	Intervet Pvt. Ltd (Merck Animal Health)	Livestock	FMD, HS, BQ, Brucellosis, Clostridium
9.	Merial Animal Health (A Sanofi Company)	Small ruminants	Clostridium

4.1.3 Disease Profiles and Epidemiology

Livestock population in India is threatened by periodic disease outbreaks, droughts, floods and other climatic anomalies. Several livestock diseases affect the

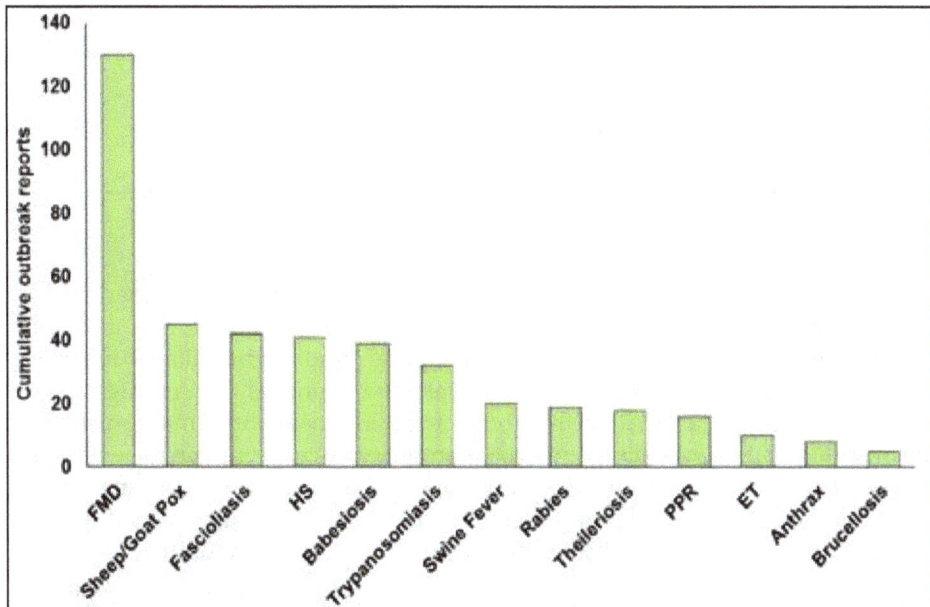

Figure 4.8: Economically Important Livestock Diseases.

Source: National Institute for Veterinary Epidemiology and Disease Informatics (NIVEDI).

sector with devastating impact on the animal productivity, production, trade and the overall economic development in Figure 4.8. The prevalent diseases to which livestock are vulnerable are categorized as bacterial, viral and parasitic diseases as described in Table 4.4. Endemic livestock diseases are likely to be the single largest cause of financial loss in the country's agriculture, and adversely affect animal welfare and trade. Foot and mouth disease is the most economically important disease in livestock followed by sheep and goat pox.

Table 4.4: Prevalent Livestock Diseases in India

Bacterial Diseases	Anthrax
	Black Quarter (BQ)
	Enterotoxaemia
	Contagious Caprine Pleuro Pneumonia (CCPP)
	Hemorrhagic Septicemia (HS)
	Brucellosis
	Foot Rot
	Botulism
Viral Diseases	Blue Tongue
	Classical Swine Fever (CSF)
	Foot and Mouth Disease (FMD)
	Peste des Petits Ruminants (PPR)
	Rabies
	Sheep and Goat Pox
Parasitic Diseases	Babesiosis
	Schistomiasis
	Theileriosis
	Paramphistomiasis
	Fasciolosis

4.1.4 Surveillance

The animal disease surveillance in the developed countries is undertaken by government by several robust national programs aided by satellite monitoring for the prevalent and most susceptible diseases in the regions. Surveillance initiatives by public-private partnership in a few developing countries such as Afghanistan have proven to be efficient in formulating various disease control mechanisms. On the other hand, the surveillance in India is an active system wherein the veterinary authority actively searches for disease evidence through survey of farmers using questionnaire, participatory surveillance tools, serological surveys and abattoir observations and samples collected and tested in diagnostic laboratory.

In India, the Project Directorate on animal disease monitoring and surveillance (PD-ADMAS), now National Institute of Veterinary Epidemiology and Disease Informatics (NIVEDI) setup under the regulations of Indian Council of Agricultural

Research (ICAR), caters to the need of surveillance and monitoring of livestock diseases. The institute has been delivering predicted informatics and solutions for various animal diseases through various activities and has developed a web portal NADRES which will forecast the probability of the occurrence of a diseases in a particular district, two months in advance. The livestock population and disease profiles are available in the databank of the institute and various departments of the institute work towards designing of various forecasting and forewarning modules in order to predict the livestock disease outbreaks. There is negligible surveillance activity carried out by the private players for the livestock sector and the surveillance reports submitted by the private organizations for renewal of the manufacturing and distribution licenses are not publicly available.

4.1.5 Vaccination Programs and Practices

Vaccination Schedules

The ICAR recommends the below vaccination schedule for the livestock animal in the country (Table 4.5). Though the recommended schedule is widely practiced, some vaccinations are given more periodically based on diseases endemicity and risk of exposure to the pathogens (Table 4.6).

Vaccine	Primary Vaccination	Booster	Revaccination
Cattle and Buffalo			
FMD vaccine	6 - 8 wks of age	6 months after 1st dose	Annually
HS vaccine	6 months and above	—	Annually
BQ vaccine	6 months and above	—	Annually
Anthrax vaccine	6 months and above	—	Annually in endemic areas
Brucella vaccine	4-8 months female calf	—	—
Swine			
Vaccine	Primary vaccination	Booster	Revaccination
CSF vaccine	2 months and above	6 months after 1st dose	Annually
FMD vaccine	2 months and above	6 months after 1st dose	Every 6 months
Sheep and Goat			
Vaccine	Primary vaccination	Booster	Revaccination
FMD vaccine	4 months and above	6 months after 1st dose	Annually
ET vaccine	4 - 6 wks of age	2 - 3 wks after 1st dose	Every 6 months
HS vaccine	6 months and above	—	Annually
CCPP vaccine	6 months and above	—	Annually
PPR vaccine	4 months and above	—	Every 3 yrs
Pox vaccine	4 months and above	—	Annually
BQ vaccine	6 months and above	—	Annually

Source: ICAR, KIRAN (Knowledge Innovation Repository of Agriculture in the North East).

Table 4.5: Demand Estimation of Livestock Vaccines

Vaccine	Animal Type	No. of Animals (in millions)	Vaccine/Year Requirement	Demand Based on Population (in millions)	Demand Based on disease Endemicity (in millions)	Total Supply (in millions)	Per cent Unmet Demand
FMD	Bovines	299	2	600	479	450	
FMD	Sheep, Goat	200	2	400.4	320	0	100
FMD	Swine	10.3	2	20.5	16.6	0	100
HS+BQ	Bovines	299	1	299	299	270	46
HS+BQ	Sheep, Goat	200	1	200	200		
Anthrax	Bovines, Sheep, Goat	500	1	500	23.6	Information not available	NA
Brucella*	Female bovines	216	1	216	216	Information not available	NA
Enterotoxaemia	Sheep, Goat	200	2	400	400	Information not available	NA
CCPP	Sheep, Goat	200	1	200	–	Information not available	NA
PPR	Sheep, Goat	200	0.33	67	38	Information not available	NA
Pox	Sheep, Goat	200	1	200	200	Information not available	NA
CSF	Swine	10.3	2	20.6	4.9	1.2	75.3

* Brucella vaccination is carried out for female bovine population only.

Table 4.6: Vaccination Schedule for different Animals

Sl.No.	Disease	Animal	Vaccine	Dose	Immunity	Time of Vaccination
1	Foot and Mouth Diseases (FMD)	All cloven footed animals	Polyvalent FMD vaccine	3 ml. S/C	1 Year	February and December
2	Hemorrhagic Septicemia (HS)	Cattle, Buffalo	HS Vaccine	5 ml S/C	6 month and 1 year	May-June
3	Black Quarter(BQ)	Cattle, Buffalo	BQ Vaccine	5 ml S/C	6 month and 1 year	May-June
4	Anthrax	All species of animals	Anthrax spore vaccine	1 ml S/C	1 Year	May-June
5	Enterotoxemia (ET)	Sheep and Goat	ET Vaccine	5 ml S/C	1 Year	May-June
6	Contagious Caprine Pleuro Pneumonia (CCPP)	Sheep and Goat	IVRI Vaccine	0.2 ml S/C	1 Year	–
7	Peste Des Pettis Ruminants (PPR)	Sheep and Goat	PPR Vaccine	1 ml S/C	3 Year	–
8	Brucellosis	Female cattle and buffalo calf age 4-8 months only	Brucella Vaccine	2 ml S/C	1 Year	–
9	Theileriosis	Cattle and calves above 2 months of age	Theileria Vaccine	3 ml S/C	1 Year	–
10	Rabies	All species of animals	Rabies Post Bite Vaccine	1 ml S/C	1 Year	0, 3,7,14,28 and 90 days

Source: Department of animal husbandry Madhya Pradesh website.

Though the disease prevalence varies across global animal populations, the vaccination schedules in the developed countries significantly cover major diseases with vaccination schedules included for the least prevalent diseases as preventive measures with appropriate notifiable steps and recognition in the immunization programs and diseases (Table 4.7). Good vaccination practices and management would lead to better animal health with increased productivity and profitability through disease prevention.

Table 4.7: OIE-Listed Diseases, Infections and Infestations in Force in 2015

Sl.No.	Species	Diseases
1.	Multiple species diseases, infections and infestations	☆ Anthrax
		☆ Bluetongue
		☆ Brucellosis (*Brucella abortus*)
		☆ Brucellosis (*Brucella melitensis*)
		☆ Brucellosis (*Brucella suis*)
		☆ Crimean Congo haemorrhagic fever
		☆ Epizootic haemorrhagic disease
		☆ Equine encephalomyelitis (Eastern)
		☆ Foot and mouth disease
		☆ Heartwater
		☆ Infection with Aujeszky's disease virus
		☆ Infection with *Echinococcus granulosus*
		☆ Infection with *Echinococcus multilocularis*
		☆ Infection with rabies virus
		☆ Infection with Rift Valley fever virus
		☆ Infection with rinderpest virus
		☆ Infection with *Trichinella* spp.
		☆ Japanese encephalitis
		☆ New world screwworm (*Cochliomyia hominivorax*)
		☆ Old world screwworm (*Chrysomya bezziana*)
		☆ Paratuberculosis
		☆ Q fever
		☆ Surra (*Trypanosoma evansi*)
		☆ Tularemia
		☆ West Nile fever
2.	Sheep and goat diseases and infections	☆ Caprine arthritis/encephalitis
		☆ Contagious agalactia
		☆ Contagious caprine pleuropneumonia
		☆ Infection with *Chlamydophila abortus* (Enzootic abortion of ewes, ovine chlamydiosis)
		☆ Infection with peste des petits ruminants virus
		☆ Maedi-visna

Contd...

Table 4.7—*Contd...*

Sl.No.	Species	Diseases
		☆ Nairobi sheep disease
		☆ Ovine epididymitis (*Brucella ovis*)
		☆ Salmonellosis (*S. abortusovis*)
		☆ Scrapie
		☆ Sheep pox and goat pox
3.	Swine diseases and infection	☆ African swine fever
		☆ Infection with classical swine fever virus
		☆ Nipah virus encephalitis
		☆ Porcine cysticercosis
		☆ Porcine reproductive and respiratory syndrome
		☆ Transmissible gastroenteritis
4.	Cattle diseases and infections	☆ Bovine anaplasmosis
		☆ Bovine babesiosis
		☆ Bovine genital campylobacteriosis
		☆ Bovine spongiform encephalopathy
		☆ Bovine tuberculosis
		☆ Bovine viral diarrhoea
		☆ Enzootic bovine leukosis
		☆ Haemorrhagic septicaemia
		☆ Infectious bovine rhinotracheitis/infectious pustular vulvovaginitis
		☆ Infection with Mycoplasma mycoides subsp. mycoides SC (Contagious bovine pleuropneumonia)
		☆ Lumpy skin disease
		☆ Theileriosis
		☆ Trichomonosis
		☆ Trypanosomosis (tsetse-transmitted)
5.	Avian diseases and infections	☆ Avian chlamydiosis
		☆ Avian infectious bronchitis
		☆ Avian infectious laryngotracheitis
		☆ Avian mycoplasmosis (*Mycoplasma gallisepticum*)
		☆ Avian mycoplasmosis (*Mycoplasma synoviae*)
		☆ Duck virus hepatitis
		☆ Fowl typhoid
		☆ Infection with avian influenza viruses
		☆ infection with influenza A viruses of high pathogenicity in birds other than poultry including wild birds
		☆ Infection with Newcastle disease virus
		☆ Infectious bursal disease (Gumboro disease)
		☆ Pullorum disease
		☆ Turkey rhinotracheitis

Source: World organization for animal health website www.ioe.int.

Based on the above given vaccination schedule, disease endemicity surveillance data and 19th census livestock, the demand-supply analysis of vaccines for major economically importance disease has been compiled below. The analysis gives us a rough estimate of the current vaccine demand-supply scenario in the country. From the analysis, we thereby conclude that the current National FMD vaccination program covers the entire bovine population with large supplies from companies such as IIL, Brilliant BioPharma, *etc.* fulfilling the entire demand of the country. The FMD program does not cover small ruminants and swine population and hence there is a 100 per cent unmet seen in this sector for FMD. Furthermore, an unmet demand for HS, BQ and CSF vaccine is observed which are manufactured and supplied by the public institutions which necessitate private players to fulfill the gap.

4.2 Poultry Biologicals Industry

Population

The poultry industry in India had risen from a mere backyard operation to a fastest growing industry with an annual turnover of USD 7.9 billion (INR 350 billion) and growing at a rate of 12-15 per cent annually [Vibrant Gujarat 2013, Government of Gujarat Report]. India emerged as the fifth largest egg producer in the world (after China and the United States of America), and eighteenth largest broiler producer [FAO reports]. This impressive growth is a due to vibrant private sector participation, integration of supply chain, geographically consolidated markets and international technology access. Increased domestic consumption of poultry products primarily led broilers to grow at greater than 10 per cent and layers at 5 – 6 per cent. Poultry provides employment to more than 3 million people, mostly women, delivers economical protein, assists in malnutrition reduction and poverty alleviation [India.gov.in, Archives].

According to 2012 census, 12.4 per cent population growth rate was observed which is significantly lower than the previous 2007 census due to the bird flu scare which led to decreased product consumption as well as decreased exports to neighboring countries. The industry still recorded a significant growth with the ability to recuperate due to effective management practices and awareness amongst farmers. The industry today is supported by a broad and strong genetic base in which the productivity levels of broilers and layers are equal to those achieved elsewhere (*e.g.* in the United States of America and the European Union) (Figure 4.9) [The poultry industry in India, FAO]. Venkateshwara group's layer breed BV 300 and broiler breed Vencobb 400 dominates the Indian poultry industry (Table 4.8).

Overview of the Poultry Industry Structure

The poultry industry has grown largely due to private sector's initiative with considerable support from the complementary veterinary health, poultry feed, equipment and processing sectors. The organized sector contributes to nearly 70 per cent of the total output and large scale producers Venkateshwara Hatcheries and Suguna Poultry Limited account for a large share of the output as they incorporate all aspects of production, including the raising of grandparent and parent flocks, rearing DOCs, contracting production, compounding feed, providing veterinary

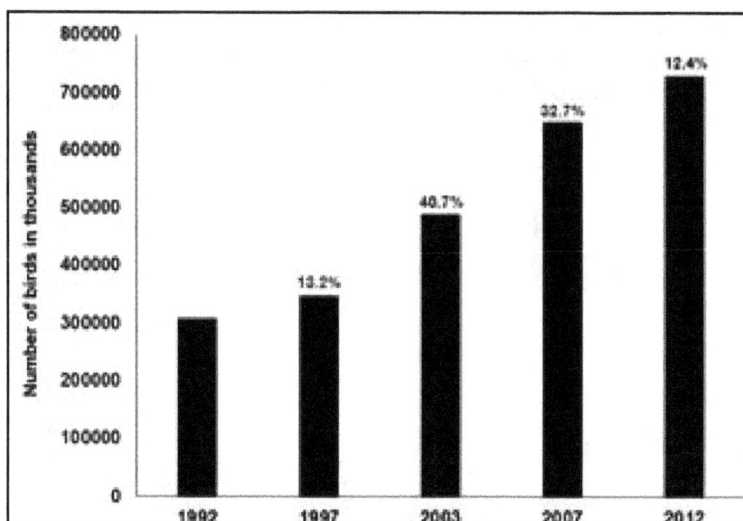

Figure 4.9: Poultry Population Census.

services, and commercial marketing of products. The rest 30 per cent is in the unorganized sector and comprises of several fragmented small farms and backyard poultry. The industry has experienced high level of consolidation over the years with the two dominant players getting stronger and the industry evolving into a highly oligopolistic one. Moreover, these dominant players have developed high level of vertical integration and are engaged in production of various inputs required for the industry as well as in strengthening market presence including front end branded products and food service.

Table 4.8: Vision 2020 for the Indian Poultry Industry

Segment/Parameter	Year 2005	Year 2010	Year 2020
Breeders	11 mil.	18 mil.	30 mil.
Layers	140 mil.	230 mil.	350 mil.
No. of broilers	1,440 mil.	2,400 mil.	3,900 mil.
Broiler meat (tonnes)	2.5	4	7.6
Employment	2.0 mil.	2.8 mil.	3.7 mil.

Source: All India Poultry Breeders Association, Industry Sources.

Average poultry farm size is getting bigger (Broiler farm – 10,000 and Layer Farm – 10,000) and productivity metrics (Feed Conversion Ratio (FCR) 1.65 – 1.70, 300 – 320 eggs per bird) are closing gap with developed nations. Biosecurity practices, environment control practices (temp and humidity), automation and mechanization are emerging to be adopted at the poultry farm to improve performance. Major MNCs have scientific and technical collaboration with leading domestic firms to access their markets. There is significant variation in the industry across regions with concentrated pockets as the broiler industry being well dominated by the southern states in our country with nearly 60-70 per cent total output coming from these states as shown in Figure 4.10. The layer industry once again is represented more in Andhra Pradesh, Tamil Nadu and Maharashtra producing nearly 70 per cent of the country's egg production.

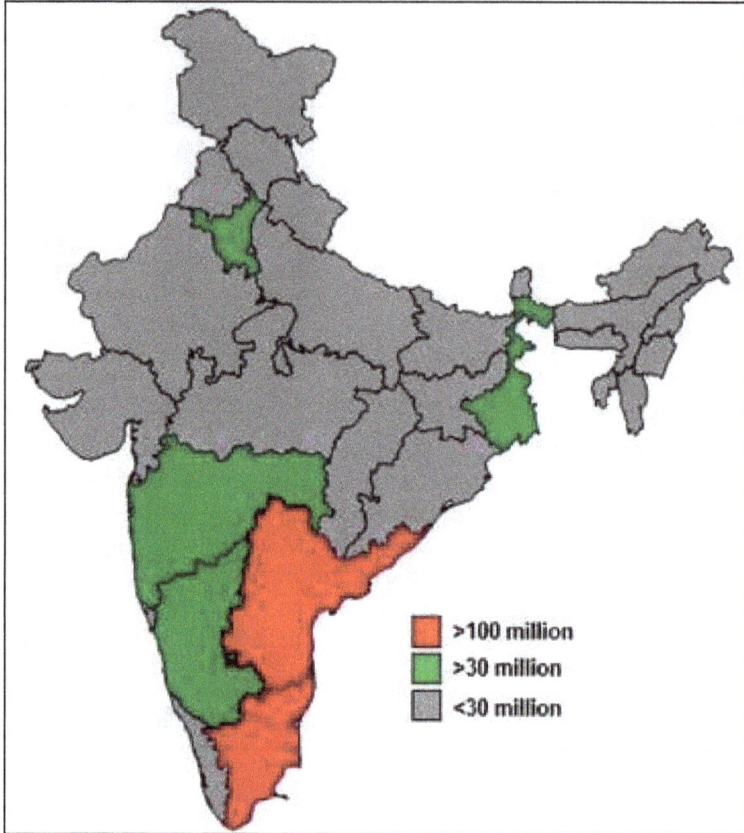

Figure 4.10: Poultry Population Clusters in India.

As mentioned earlier, poultry plays a very important part in Indian economy with eggs and chicken meat being rich sources of protein. Chicken is the most widely accepted meat in India. Unlike beef or pork, it does not have any religious sentiments attached to it and is comparatively cheaper than goat meat or mutton, thereby easily available to people. In the last two to three decades, poultry has made tremendous strides particularly in the private sector, with the result that India is now self-sufficient with regard to requirements of high quality breeding stocks, modern poultry equipment, availability of medicines and vaccines and technically qualified skilled manpower. The Indian poultry meat is majorly domestically consumed and exported to neighboring countries like Nepal and Bangladesh with export volumes being very low (Figure 4.11) [Agri Export Advantage, EXIM Bank Report March 2014]. A fluctuating market is seen in exports due to uncertainty in regulations

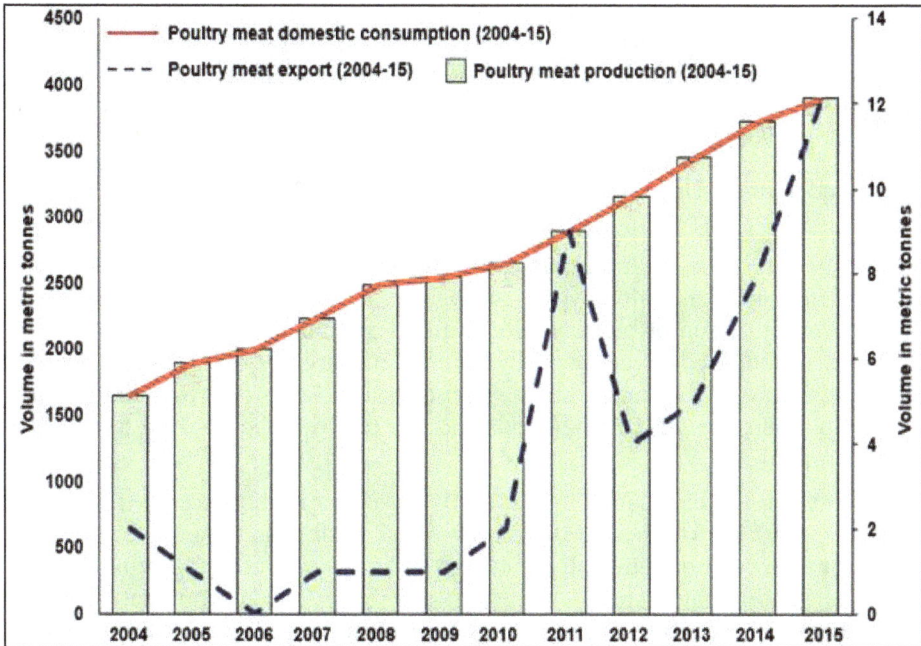

Figure 4.11: Trends in Poultry Meat Production, Domestic Consumption and Export.
Source: **USDA.**

and various disease outbreaks. The outbreak of avian influenza in 2007-08 caused a decrease in the rate of production along with stagnant exports.

The annual growth rate is 8-10 per cent in egg and 12-15 per cent in the broiler industry. With the annual production of 33 billion eggs, India is the fifth world's largest egg producing country. It also produces 530 million broilers per year. This is much lower as compared to the world average of 124 eggs and 5.9 kg meat. The National Committee on Human Nutrition in India has recommended per capita of 180 eggs (about one egg every two days) and 10.8 kg meat. To meet this target, it is estimated that by year 2010, the requirements will be 180 billion eggs and 9.1 billion kg poultry meat while the estimated production may only be around 46.2 billion eggs and 3.04 billion kg poultry meat. This shows that there is a tremendous scope for growth with rapid urbanization, and increasing demand from the present 250 million economically strong, consumer market base, there is bright future for this industry in India.

Given the derivative demand directly linked to the poultry industry, the poultry vaccine industry has experienced the same trends with respect to high historical growth rate and promising industry outlook. Considering the significant consolidation and corporate interest in the poultry industry, the commercial motive behind decision making is high. The industry recognizes the commercial implication of potential losses due to disease outbreaks and the importance of vaccination. Vaccination practices are widely adopted and followed. Consequently, the poultry vaccines market is a relatively more commercially attractive segment within veterinary vaccines and is largely a private market with no substantial public procurement. However, it tends to be a difficult market for new companies to break into as elaborated further below in our analysis of level of competition using the Porter's Five Forces framework.

Complexity of an Oligopolistic Industry with high Vertical Integration

Concentrated buyer power and high barrier to entry: As described earlier, significant part of the poultry industry is part of the organized sector that is heavily consolidated and dominated by two companies, Venky's and Suguna. This results in high concentration of buyer power in these dominant players. In addition to wielding concentrated buyer power, these companies are highly vertically integrated and have their own vaccine production capabilities. Hence, they are often capable of meeting their own vaccine demands and this proves to be a barrier to entry for other companies.

Ventri Biologicals setup in the early seventies is the vaccine division of Venkateshwara Hatcheries (VH) Group which has diverse stakes in breeding of poultry, poultry equipment, hatcheries, egg and chicken processing, animal health products, production of specific pathogen free (SPF) eggs and poultry feed. This vaccine division was one of the initial poultry vaccine manufacturers in the country set up at a time when the Indian Poultry Industry was facing severe challenges due to unavailability of quality vaccines for several disease conditions. Globion India Pvt. Ltd. is a joint venture between Suguna Holdings Private Limited, and German-based Lohmann Animal Health GmbH, to produce vaccines primarily for poultry. It started its pre-operation activities from 2006, and started full operations as of 2010 and produces both live and inactivated vaccines. The company is the largest producer of New Castle disease vaccine, both live and inactivated; manufacturing 1000 million doses annually (Figure 4.12).

1. MNCs and R&D driven Indian vaccine companies leverage portfolio strengths to break barrier to entry

Other key players in the industry (Table 4.9) have leveraged their portfolio strengths to establish themselves in this market by filling product portfolio gaps of the industry leaders. This includes multinational companies (such as Merial, Intervet and Zoetis) that have the advantage of drawing from their global product portfolio and R&D strength and Indian companies such as Hester and Indovax that have leveraged specialized vaccines to break the entry barrier created by vertically integrated industry leaders who control buyer power. An example of such a product includes the recombinant vaccine for Marek's disease (Merck and Hester Pharmaceuticals Ltd). Additionally, companies such as Hester are also trying to reach the backyard poultry market and gain share in the remaining 30 per cent that is not controlled by the industry leaders. The public institutions run by the State Governments produce the vaccines for the most prevalent diseases in the region for backyard poultry too with their internal supply chain and distribution channels.

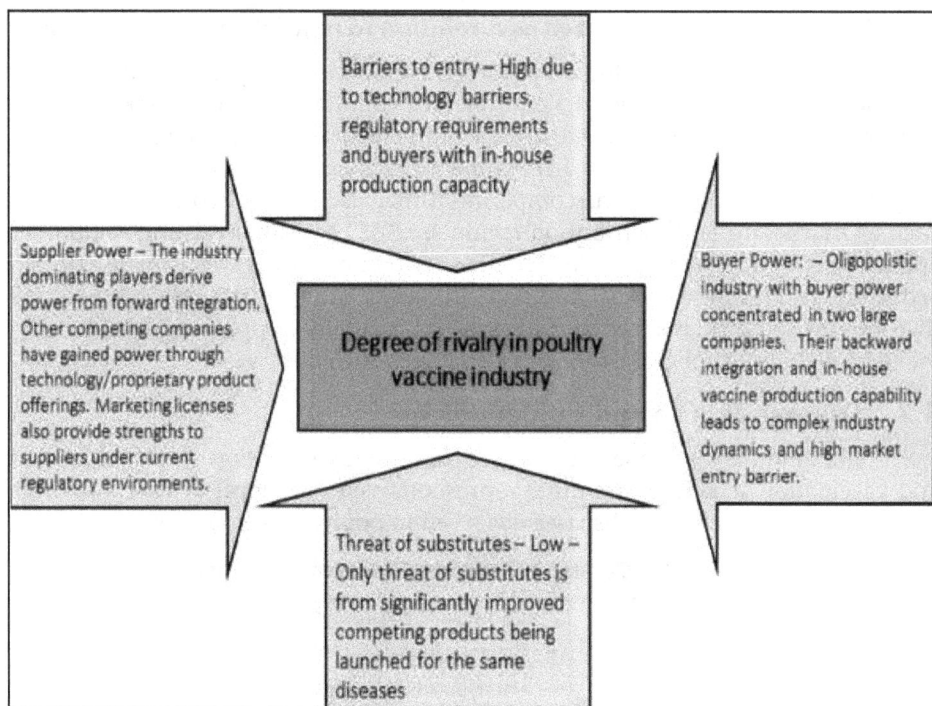

Figure 4.12: Overview of the Poultry Vaccine Industry.

Table 4.9: Key Players in the Indian Poultry Vaccine

Sl.No.	Organization	Vaccine Products
1.	Biomed	Bursal Disease, Newcastle, Bronchitis, Fowl Pox, Marek's Disease
2.	Globion India Pvt. Limited	Newcastle, Bronchitis, Fowl pox
3.	Hester Biosciences Ltd	Bursal Disease, Newcastle, Bronchitis, Coryza, Reo virus, Fowl Cholera, Fowl Pox, Egg drop syndrome, Herpes.
4.	Indovax Private Limited	Bursal Disease, Newcastle, Bronchitis, Coryza, Reo virus, Fowl pox, Marek's Disease
5.	Intervet Pvt. Ltd (Merck Animal Health)	Bursal disease, Mycoplasma, Newcastle, Bronchitis, Coryza, Reo virus, Salmonellosis
6.	Merial Animal Health (A Sanofi Company)	Bursal, Mycoplasma, Newcastle, Bronchitis, Coryza, Reo virus, Salmonella, Fowl pox, Marek's Disease, Egg drop syndrome, Swollen Head Syndrome, Viral Arthritis
7.	Ventri Biologicals	Bursal, Newcastle, Bronchitis, Marek's Disease
8.	Zoetis India Limited (Pfizer Animal Health)	Bursal, Mycoplasma, Newcastle, Bronchitis, Coryza, Reo virus, Marek's Disease
9.	Zydus Animal Health	Bursal disease, Newcastle, Bronchitis, Coryza, Fowl Cholera, Viral Arthritis

2. Collaborations being pursued as a solution to regulatory barriers to entry

In the past decade, the Indian poultry vaccines and diagnostic manufactures have witnessed a number joint ventures and collaborations for marketing and distribution of their products. Due to enormous constraints and delays in obtaining regulatory approvals, short lifespan of poultry biologicals (8-10 years due to evolving nature of poultry diseases), the companies utilize each other's core competencies such as marketing and distribution channels, R&D pipeline, existing regulatory approvals *etc*. One such example M&A is Dosch Pharmaceuticals Private Limited acquired by Merial, a Sanofi company to enter India. With Dosch's existing distribution network, marketing channels and regulatory approvals, Merck could make its global portfolio of products available in the country.

4.2.1 Disease Profile and Epidemiology

Poultry industry is one segment where preventive vaccination is well established and vaccination schedules are quite representative of the local disease situation. Following are the common diseases observed in poultry given in Table 4.10.

Table 4.10: Common Diseases Observed in Poultry

Bacterial Diseases	Escherichia coli infections
	Salmonellosis
	Paratyphoid infections
	Fowl cholera
	Riemerella anatipestifer infections
	Mycoplasma
	Necrotic enteritis
	Cholangiohepatitis in broiler chickens
	Gangrenous dermatitis
	Avian tuberculosis
Neoplastic Diseases	Virus-induced neoplastic diseases Marek's
	Lymphoid leucosis
	Myelocytomatosis
	Erythroblastosis
	Adenocarcinomatosis
	Botulism
Parasitic Diseases	Coccidiosis
	Histomonosis
	Ascaridiosis
	Raillietinosis
	Knemidokoptosis
Mycoses and Mycotoxicoses	Aspergillosis
	Aspergillus granulomatous dermatitis

Contd...

Table 4.10–*Contd...*

	Aflatoxicosis
	Candidiasis
	Fusariotoxicoses
Viral Diseases	Viral inclusion body hepatitis
	Hemorrhagic enteritis of turkeys
	Egg drop syndrome -1976
	Adenovirus group i -associated infections
	Infectious bursal disease (Gumboro)
	Infectious bronchitis (IB)
	Laryngotracheitis
	Swollen head syndrome
	Infectious encephalomyelitis
	Newcastle disease
	Fowl pox
	Reo Virus infections

Newcastle disease is the most prevalent disease in the avian population followed by Coccidiosis, Fowl Pox, IBD, Fowl Cholera, Marek's Disease, Salmonellosis (Figure 4.13) as per the number of disease outbreaks reported (Annual report 2014-15, DADF).

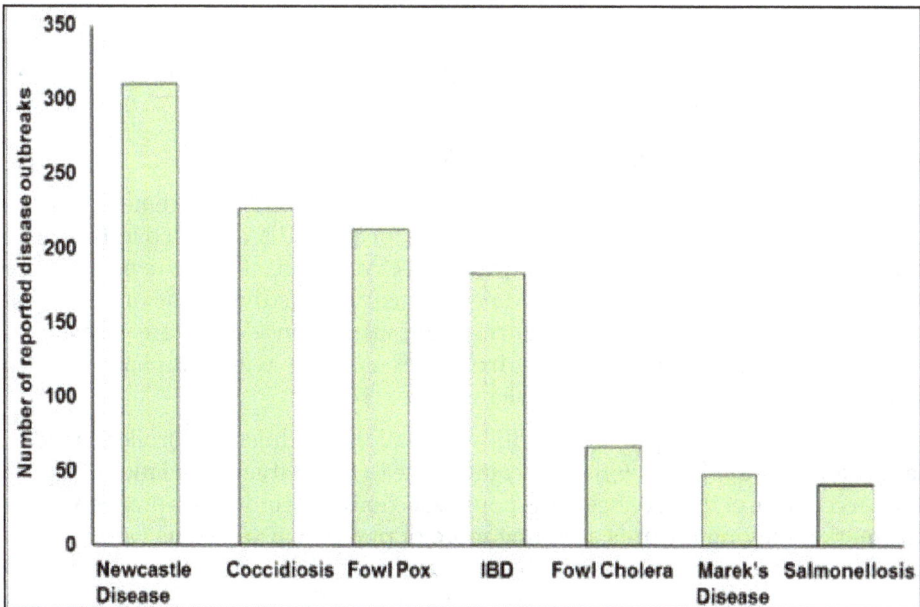

Figure 4.13: Prevalent Diseases in Poultry.

4.2.2 Surveillance

India is self-sufficient in all basic equipment that is required for rearing and breeding poultry with support from all nationalized and commercial banks in the country to provide facilities to invest in poultry ventures. In spite of the tremendous progress made in developing diagnostics and vaccines, serious problems still exist with respect to disease surveillance and monitoring because of lack of adequate infrastructure.

The diseases surveillance in the poultry sector is done in majority by a few organizations and has been intensified since 2001 with the surveillance for Avian influenza and has been further strengthened with the incorporation of High Security Animal Disease Laboratory (HSADL) now renamed as ICAR- National Institute of High Security Animal Diseases, Bhopal for the purpose of both diagnosis and surveillance and intensified surveillance of Avian Influenza in poultry farms located near or around water bodies/sanctuaries identified by the Ministry of Environment and Forests with the visit of migratory/wild birds for their winter nesting. The poultry surveillance with non-infectious antigens is also being taken up with five regional disease diagnostic laboratories under the DADF. Poultry Diagnostic and Research Centers of Ventri Biologicals is one private organization which provides technical service and carries disease surveillance across the country along with other private vaccine manufacturing organizations as a compliance for renewing the manufacturing, marketing and distribution license of respective vaccines of the diseases recognized by Government of India. These surveillance reports are submitted to the regulatory body and are not publicly available. While there is no data publicly available surveillance data, there is also lack of information on the poultry disease incidence in the country. The sector seeks surveillance data with epidemiology information of the seasonal influenza since the vaccine for influenza infection is based on the circulating virus strains and the country has to strengthen monitoring mechanisms.

4.2.3 Vaccination Schedules and Practices

Vaccination schedule depends on type of bird, regional requirement, disease prevalence and breed's susceptibility. Vaccines for all the diseases cited in Table 4.11 are produced by both the public and private sector in India with more prominence of the private sector for the consolidated industry while the public organization majorly supply to the backyard poultry. Public institutions do prepare vaccination schedules for backyard poultry but have serious issues with compliance. These institutions do cover the most prevalent disease, NDV.

Private companies prepare specific vaccination schedules *e.g.* (broiler, breeder, layer etc) and administer with high compliance to their target population. There is high acceptance of the vaccines in the poultry section as the industry's preference and the market moving towards adopting more of prevention strategies (vaccination) as cost of treatment/diagnosis is high and non-existent. The vaccines prepared in private sector are produced with the use of Specific Pathogen Free (SPF) eggs but the same may not be true with public institutions. According to FAO reports, vaccines manufactured for poultry in India meet international standards and prices of these vaccines, animal health products and food additives are either comparable or slightly higher than international prices.

Table 4.11: Vaccination Schedule

Days	Vaccine	Route
Layer Birds		
1-3 days	Gumboro (intermediate) vaccine	Eye drop
7 days	Lasota vaccine	Eye drop
14 days	Gumboro (intermediate) vaccine (repeat)	Eye drop
18 days	Mareks disease vaccine	0.2 ml by intramuscular or subcutaneous injection
21-23 days	Infectious bronchitis vaccine + Lasota as combined vaccine	Drinking water
28-30 days	Gumboro (intermediate) vaccine (repeat)	Drinking water
42 days	Fowl pox vaccine	Wing web prick(stab)
Week 8	Lasota vaccine (repeat) Infectious coryza (bacterin)	Drinking water Intramuscular injection
Week 11-12	Infectious bronchitis + Lasota as combined vaccine (Repeat)	Drinking water
Week 13	Ranikhet disease vaccine (R2B)	Intramuscular injection
Week 14	Fowl pox vaccine (repeat) if necessary	Wing web prick
Week 18	Ranikhet disease vaccine (killed)	Subcutaneous injection
Broiler Birds		
6-7 days	Ranikhet disease (F1 OR B1)	Eye drop or nasal drop
10-12 days	Gumboro (intermediate)	Drinking water
18-21 days	Lasota vaccine(intermediate)	Drinking water
24-30 days	Gumboro disease (intermediate)	Drinking water

These poultry vaccines require high degree of precision and accuracy along with stringent standards for producing the right kind of vaccines to combat the highly mutagenic pathogens and most prevalent diseases in the poultry industry. However, we understand from interaction with industry that there are concerns around surveillance practices and recognition of existence of certain diseases and consequently these are not covered under the current vaccination schedule.

Two examples noted from interactions are avian influenza where lack of recognition in surveillance has led to informal trade of vaccines and the globally most pathogenic strain of Marek's disease vaccination given as a preventive measure is still not included in the Indian vaccination schedule.

4.2.4 Drivers and Opportunities

1. Emerging Diseases

Poultry has short generation interval among the production animals and needs to be reproduced continually. Vaccinations are essential against dangerous pathogens and the host immunity continuously exerts selection pressure on pathogens. Viral RNA genomes are susceptible to point mutations during replication. One estimate indicates point mutations as high as one per million in 12 hr replication. Hence, mutations lead to new viral strains and emerging diseases such as different NDV genotypes, IBD virus mutants, IB variants *etc.*

High susceptibility of commercial birds, pathogen's evolving genetic profile, role of migratory birds that bring in the new pathogens from other parts of the globe cause emergence of new avian diseases. The avian pathogens from these emerging diseases, are highly mutagenic that affects lifespan of the poultry vaccines. Typically, poultry vaccine lifespan is around 8-10 years while that of livestock vaccine lifespan is over 40 -50 years. Vaccination and medication, coupled with strict biosecurity measures, are needed to prevent the spread of these diseases. There exists further opportunities for poultry vaccine manufacturers on recognition of certain diseases that are currently not declared in the country such as infectious laryngotracheitis, chicken anemia, infectious bronchitis and Marek's disease variants. With recognition of prevalence of these strains, there exists a need to develop vaccines in short duration which would further prevent informal trade and practices for these diseases vaccinations. Though the Indian poultry segment has the product development capacity, the availability of vaccines is delayed due to ineffective disease reporting mechanism and suppressed reporting in several occasions which hinders accelerated approval mechanism during disease outbreaks

2. Increasing Population and Global Consumption

In 2012, global consumption of broiler meat is 13.6 kg per capita per annum and 9 kg (170 – 180 eggs) per capita per annum. Indian Consumption of broiler meat is 2.8 kg per capita per annum and 55 eggs per capita per annum. Indian eggs consumption is much lower when compared to the world average (in 2002, Mexico-321, USA- 255, France-248, Portugal-186) [International Egg Commission]. Indian broiler meat consumption is much lower to other leading countries (in 2011, USA – 43.81, Australia – 43.66, Brazil – 39.94, Peru -37.45) [International Poultry Council].

The National Committee on Human Nutrition in India has recommended per capita of 180 eggs (about one egg every two days) and 10.8 kg meat. With greater acceptance of eggs as an important source of proteins, vitamins and minerals and broiler chicken being the most widely accepted meat in India, there has been a significant increase of domestic consumption of poultry products. India's changing eating habits, rising purchasing power, and increasing urbanization is likely to sustain continued growth in demand and consumption of poultry products. The increase in demand has led to an increase in the bird population with large corporate, thereby triggering a demand for the vaccines for the wellbeing of the birds.

3. Backyard Poultry

A GALVmed commissioned study showed that India has two highly polarized poultry vaccine markets consisting of large-scale commercial integrated sector and unorganized backyard poultry sector with low vaccine coverage. Three main reasons for poor coverage of backyard poultry birds are lack of farmer awareness, inadequate rural infrastructure for cold chain management and very limited manpower with one vet or paravet managing about 25-30 villages.

Public sector supply chain caters mostly to the needs of the state poultry farms and to a very small extent, the backyard poultry sector that is unexplored by private vaccine manufacturers requiring higher distribution channels. Despite low coverage, government officials and veterinarians at all levels in the chain realized the immense importance of vaccination for the backyard poultry sector and the report estimates the backyard poultry biologicals industry at around 260 million doses of vaccine a year. Our observations suggests that willingness to pay is not an issue for the small-scale poultry keepers due to higher treatment costs in comparison to vaccination, but doorstep delivery of services is a major constraint as they are skeptical about government-provided services which are in short supply and irregular.

4.2.5 Challenges and Restraint

1. Oligopolistic Industry Structure, Barrier for New Entrants

As the poultry industry is highly consolidated, it has entry barrier for new vaccine players, as the buying power is consolidated with few companies that have high level of backward integration and have their own vaccine production arms. Despite this market entry barrier, Hester and Indovax have sustained and made their presence in the industry due to their specialty products which fill the product portfolios of the large players of the industry. While this strategy has driven commercial success for these companies until now, this might not be a sustainable strategy for new companies entering the market in near future due to saturated market presence by these companies.

2. Supply Chain Constrains

A major constraint affecting the growth of the poultry vaccines industry is limited storage and transportation infrastructure such as cold chain, that result in high cost distribution cost, low rural vaccine supply, vaccine failure and price fluctuation of the poultry products.

3. Recognition of Pathogens and Immunization Practices

Another major challenge of the industry is the lack of effective surveillance that leads to informal practices of manufacturing the vaccines by conventional methods for disease prevention without scientific documentation. Though the Research and Development for poultry vaccine is adequate to meet new disease vaccination demand with no adoption barrier of technology in the poultry sector, appropriate disclosure of the disease prevalence and the epidemiology would also lead to further R&D and improved vaccine at appropriate time.

We believe that the concerns highlighted by the vaccine manufacturers regarding the introduction of newer vaccines in the immunization policy and the informal and often surreptitious vaccination practices could be due to the surveillance carried by the vaccine manufacturers with questionable efficacy and not by the government bodies. This further accentuates the demand for strong and efficient surveillance methods which can be used by small farmers, exporters *etc.* The transparency in the surveillance would solve a lot of the above mentioned problems and also make the vaccines available in a timely manner.

4.3 Companion Animal Biologicals Industry

Population

Companion animals, most typically dogs and cats are kept by people for companionship and a range of utilitarian purposes thereby, sharing a close relationship with their owners and playing an important role in developing communities. Market news reports mark India as an emerging market growing at 10-15 per cent annually [Euromonitor Reports] and one of the best potential pet care markets in the Asian sub-continent after Japan owing to the changing lifestyles, rise in nuclear families and double income households, which have further encouraged the growth of pet ownership in the country. The societal benefits of pet ownership and the close proximity of the relation is evident by the growing pet numbers in the growing number of nuclear family lives and their participation in institutional programs.

The number of companion animals segment is a significant part of total animals in India with a population of close to 27 million (rural and urban dog population – community and pets) in 2012. Uttar Pradesh (4.8 million), Maharashtra (2.3 million), Karnataka (1.9 million), Tamil Nadu (1.8 million) and Andhra Pradesh (1.7 million) have recorded the highest density of dog population in the country (19th livestock census). As per the estimates of the industry sources, the companion animal population is close to 33 million dogs of which 25 per cent falls under the pet population, 42-45 per cent is community population and 32 per cent are family and communities owned pets. These numbers are considerably in approximation with the 19th census data from DADF. The data available from various sources is not consistent and reliable for the stray dog and cat population and hence, the only data set used in this report for population records is from 19th livestock census (Figure 4.14). The dog population has seen a considerable drop in growth from the previous year but the spending on pets in urban and semi-urban market has seen a sharp increase with an annual appending of INR 4000-5000 (as per industry experts).

In spite of the decrease of the dog population over the previous census, the Indian pet market has been constantly on a rise and is driven by several factors such as increased number of pet adoptions, rising disposable income, change in perception towards pets, increased consumption, higher awareness of dietary needs of pets and the benefits of pet food and a growing awareness towards animal and human health. Pet owners have started to take an interest in their pet's diet, health and grooming and a gradual shift towards prepared pet food has been observed. Pet owners are more willing to spend on pet food and pet care products than ever before. This trend has spawning the entire industry, with a growing emphasis on pet care.

With most of the pet food being imported and the government's reduction of the import duties on pet food in 2007 provided a boost to both manufacturers and

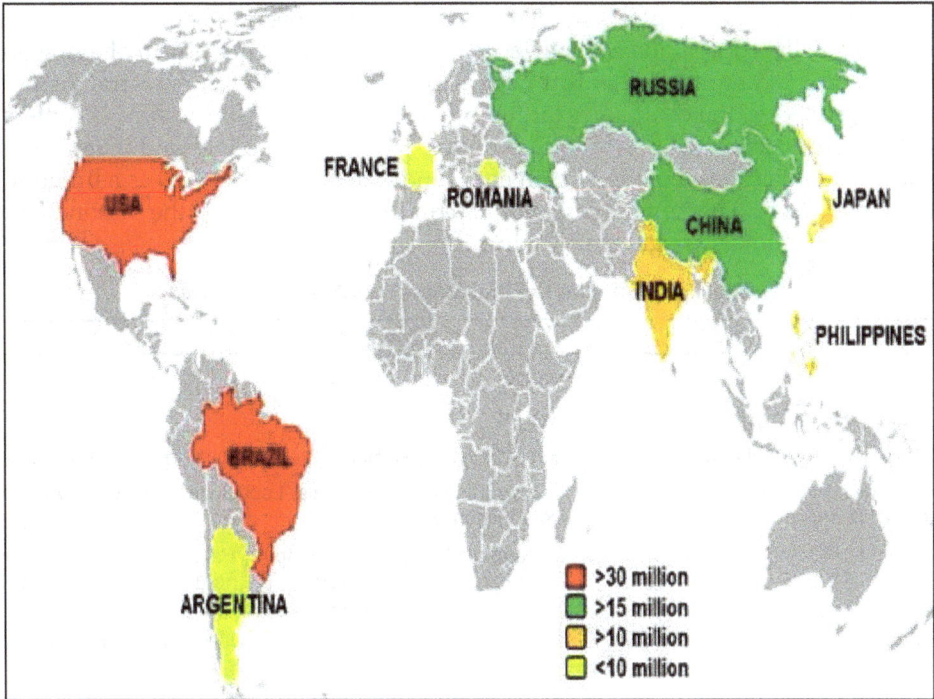

Figure 4.14: Global Companion Animal Population.

importers. But the ban on imported pet food due to the outbreak of Avian Flu in year 2006, which continued through 2007, resulted in the reduced availability of pet food. This led to an increase in local manufacturing and with reduced brand loyalty of customers; the Indian manufacturers were able to make their presence in the pet food market. Veterinary clinics and pet shops remained a leading distribution channels for pet food and pet care products till 2007 but a shift in trend towards more and more retail outlets and supermarkets started emerging as viable distribution channels. Thus, the industry has been growing at the rate of 10-15 per cent annually with the same trends to be seen in near future as well.

Companion Animal Vaccine Industry

The companion animal industry is largely dominated by pet food segment, pharmaceuticals followed by the biologicals segment. The biological products used in India and the vaccination schedules followed nationally are comparable to that of global standards. A majority of these vaccines today are imported in the country with globally prevalent strains of disease pathogens. The total companion animal market is about INR 40-60 crores and is growing at an annual rate of 10-15 per cent. Due to this comparatively small size of the market, industry experts have cited that establishing a manufacturing plant for biologicals in India might not be a financially viable decision in near future as this will require a huge capital investment followed by low revenues on sales within the country.

Majority of leading global animal healthcare companies today have made their presence in the companion animal vaccines and diagnostics in India by having an import oriented entry mechanism with established distribution network. As per industry experts, the companies target different veterinary clinics and pet centers to promote their global portfolio of products other than vaccines and diagnostics and use biological as a mode to gain entry and establish themselves as a brand in the value chain. The key players manufacturing and importing the vaccines for companion animals are given in Table 4.12.

Table 4.12: Key Players in Companion Animal Vaccines

Sl.No.	Organization	Vaccine Products
1.	Biomed	Rabies
2.	Brilliant Bio Pharm Pvt. Ltd	Rabies
3.	Indian Immunologicals Pvt. Ltd	Rabies, Distemper, Hepatitis, Leptospira, Parvovirus, Corona
4.	Intervet Pvt. Ltd (Merck Animal Health)	Rabies, Distemper, Hepatitis, Leptospira, Parvovirus, Adeno Para Influenza Virus
5.	Merial Animal Health (A Sanofi Company)	Distemper, Hepatitis, Leptospira, Parvovirus, Adeno Para Influenza Virus, Bordetella Bronchiseptica, Infectious Panleucopenia, Calcivirus Respiratory Infections
6.	Virbac Animal Health India Pvt Ltd	Rabies, Distemper, Parvo Virus, Adenovirus, Parainfluenza virus
7.	Zoetis India Limited (Pfizer Animal Health)	Rabies, Distemper, Hepatitis, Leptospira, Parvovirus, Adeno Para Influenza Virus

Due to regulatory constraints in imports and smaller market size, only few players with global portfolio strengths are active in the Indian market with lesser competition. The market shares held by the companies are not significantly different with each company owning approximately 6-10 crores of the market.

4.3.1 Disease Profiles and Epidemiology

The most prevalent canine diseases are Canine Distemper, Canine Parvo, Rabies, Kennel Cough, Leptospirosis, *Ehrlichiosis, Babesiosis etc.* which can currently be prevented and treated by various antibiotics, pharmaceuticals and vaccinations. Most of these diseases are endemic in the country with high prevalence in highly populated pocket states such as Uttar Pradesh and Maharashtra.

4.3.2 Surveillance

In spite of the tremendous growth of the companion animal industry, the disease surveillance in this sector is the least noted of all by the public sector due to least impact on the national economy. Other than the livestock population census, there is no accurate disease surveillance from public sector and similar to the poultry industry, the surveillance of companion animal diseases is conducted by the private companies and the reports are submitted to the governing bodies for compliance criteria fulfillment to obtain licenses for new vaccines or to renew older licenses for existing vaccines in the country to market and distribute biological products. These surveillance reports are not available in public domain.

4.3.3 Vaccination Programs and Practices

The current programs for companion animals run by the government are for stray animals specifically. There are no government run vaccination programs for cats but understanding the host ecology and the number of deaths in the country due to rabid dog bites which is approximately 20,000 deaths annually, the Animal Welfare Board of India (AWBI) a statutory and advisory body of the Government of India, has facilitated the implementation of street dogs rabies vaccination and sterilization called, Animal Birth Control (ABC) program. The program has been successfully impacted on control of incidence of human and animal rabies in Chennai, Jaipur, Kalimpong, Ooty and Gangktok where the programs has been implemented intensively and are now zero rabies zones. Based on this success, GOI has formulated the Dog Rules 2001 which directs that municipalities work with animal welfare organizations for implementing the ABC program is various regions (Figure 4.15). Population of companion animals as shown in Figure 4.16.

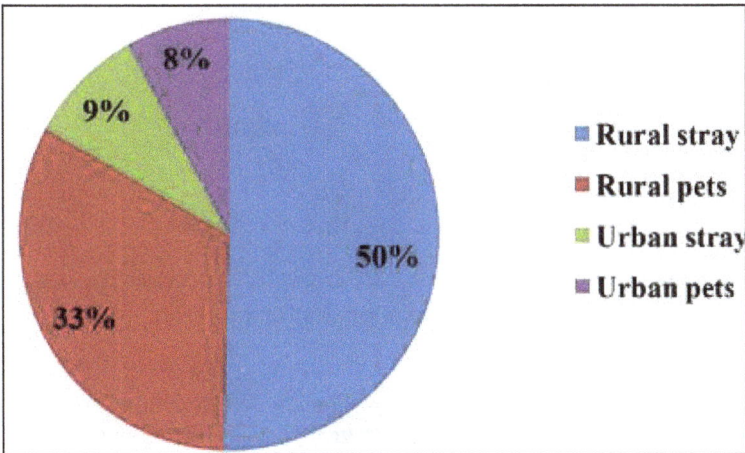

Figure 4.15: Detailed Split of Pet vs. Community Dogs.

Vaccination Schedules

Based on the above vaccination schedules Table 4.13 and Table 4.14, total value and volume of import data and total population of companion animals, an estimate of total demand-supply in the country was calculated and analyzed as depicted in the Tables 4.15 and 4.16. It was observed that an unmet demand for both combination vaccines and Rabies vaccine for pets and total dog population respectively. For the feline population of 0.35 million, which is estimated based on the estimates from industry experts, the demand was estimated with no publicly available data on vaccine supply.

4.3.4 Drivers and Opportunities

1. Growth in Overall Companion Animal Market

Industry sources indicate that the global market for companion animal health

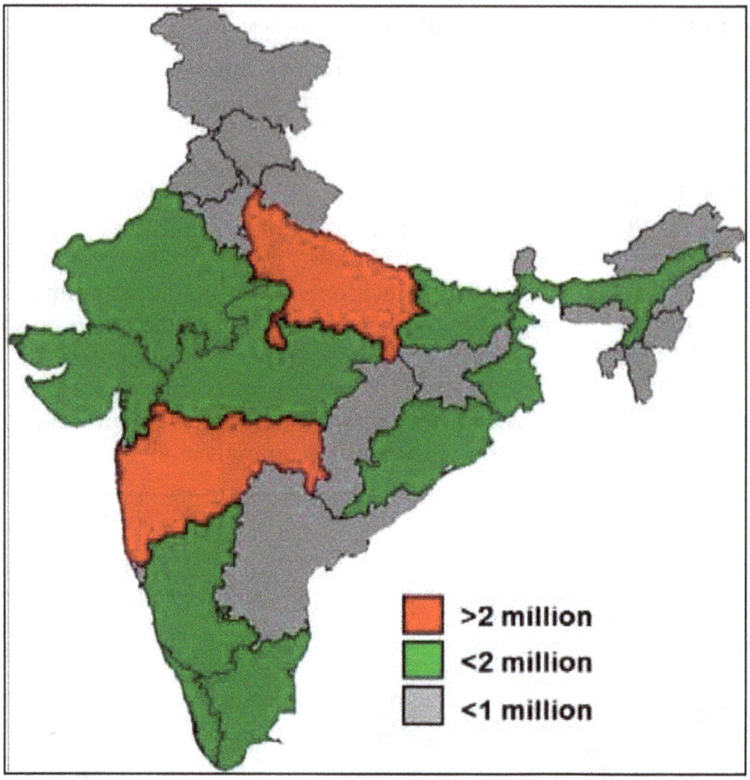

Figure 4.16: Population Distribution Map.

products is expected to further grow and become more specialized. The Indian companion animal healthcare products register a compound annual growth rate (CAGR) of 10-15 per cent. The major driver of this segment is the increase in companion animal ownership with continuous strengthening of the bond between owners and their animal companions, increase in willingness to spend for the pet animals, increased companion animal owner awareness and increasing companion animal owner demands and expectations for companion animal care. Spending on companion animals vaccines and medicines to help pets live longer, healthier lives is also continuing to increase due to economic development and related increases in disposable income in the country and is a leading driving of growth strategies of the companion animal product manufacturers.

2. Rising Awareness for Zoonotic Infections

The rise of zoonotic infections such as rabies and leptospirosis has led to increase in their prevention and control with unique practices and vaccinations coming into picture. There are various factors responsible for emergence and re-emergence of zoonotic diseases such as change in climate conditions, increased population density, increased trade, mutations etc. with the increase in awareness of zoonotic diseases amongst pet owners and community in general; there is an increased demand for

Table 4.13: Vaccination schedule of Dogs

Age	Vaccination
5 weeks	**Parvovirus**: for puppies at high risk of exposure to parvo, some veterinarians recommend vaccinating at 5 weeks.
6 and 9 weeks	**Combination vaccine** (5-way vaccine, usually includes adenovirus cough and hepatitis, distemper, parainfluenza, and parvovirus. Some combination vaccines may also include leptospirosis (7-way vaccines) and/or coronavirus without leptospirosis. **Coronavirus**: where coronavirus is a concern.
12 weeks or older	**Rabies**
12-16 weeks	**Combination vaccine** **Leptospirosis**: include leptospirosis in the combination vaccine where leptospirosis is a concern, or if traveling to an area where it occurs. **Coronavirus**: where coronavirus is a concern. **Lyme**: where Lyme disease is a concern or if traveling to an area where it occurs.
Adult (boosters)	**Combination vaccine** **Leptospirosis**: include leptospirosis in the combination vaccine where leptospirosis is a concern, or if traveling to an area where it occurs. **Coronavirus**: where coronavirus is a concern. **Lyme**: where Lyme disease is a concern or if traveling to an area where it occurs. **Rabies**: Given by your local veterinarian (time interval between vaccinations may vary according to local law).

Table 4.14: Vaccination Schedule of Cats

Age to Administer	Vaccination
8-9 weeks	FVRCP Vaccine
12 weeks	Booster Shot for FVRCP Vaccine
12 weeks	FeLV (only in cats with acute propensity, after the booster)
16 weeks	Rabies shot (if required)
1 year	Booster Shot for Rabies

Table 4.15: Demand Estimation of Canine Vaccines

Vaccine	No of Animals (in millions)	Vaccine/ Year Requirement	Total Demand (in millions)	Total Supply (in millions)	Per cent Unmet Demand
7-way combination (Adeno virus, distemper, hepatitis, parainfluenza. parvo virus, Leptospirosis, coronavirus)	11.7 (pets)	1	12	1.4	88
Rabies	27 (total dog)	1	27	15	44.44

Table 4.16: Demand Estimation of Feline Vaccines

Vaccine	No of Animals (in millions)	Vaccine/ Year Requirement	Total Demand (in millions)	Total Supply (in millions)
Feline distemper vaccine (feline rhinotracheitis)	0.15	1	0.15	NA
Calicivirus, panleukopenia) Rabies	0.35	1	0.35	NA
FeLV	0.15	1	0.15	NA

vaccines and diagnostics in the country. This could be a potential opportunity and growth driver for vaccine manufacturers to expand in near future.

3. Export Market as an Opportunity for Potential Industry Expansion

Based on our interactions with veterinary clinicians, vaccines for Kennel Cough (*Bordetella brochiseptica*), Canine Parvo and Canine Distemper are the most probable opportunities for companion animal vaccine producers to manufacture locally in India. These vaccines have a potential to be produced locally and export potential could be leveraged in future. Currently, the vaccines are imported in the country with a huge demand locally in urban and semi-urban areas with existing greater awareness on pet health. With high volumes and economies of scale in production, local manufacturing plant could be set up in future to act as a potential export hub for global demand.

4. Government Initiated National Programs

Currently, the Government of India has many national programs initiated for economically important diseases such as that in livestock (cattle and buffaloes) and small ruminants. With the implementation of these national vaccination programs, demand for livestock vaccines for diseases such as FMD, PPR, Brucellosis has risen with many small and large private players from the poultry industry entering the livestock vaccine market as an extension to their existing vaccine portfolio. With the implementation of such large scale national vaccination programs, the companion animal industry could also possibly benefit with a huge volume driver for manufacturers to enter this segment. Today, the rabies and ABC program are implemented in limited districts in the country with 100 per cent success rate in making the districts rabies free zones and this could be potentially extended nationally in near future. Thus, a future growth driver exists with the rabies vaccine and with the nationalization of the ABC program to other districts in the country thereby paving way for the entry of new players for vaccine manufacture. Manufacturers could leverage and explore the opportunities exporting companion animal vaccines with local production if the economies are viable.

4.3.5 Challenges and Restraint

1. Lack of Surveillance and Disease Epidemiology Information

A major constraint in this segment of the industry is the lack of official market data on disease prevalence and the surveillance information. There is a need to strengthen surveillance in the country and completeness of census and surveillance data for major zoonotic diseases. Due to lack of data today, we are unable to identify emerging zoonotic threats such as rabies Leptospirosis, toxoplasmosis *etc.*

2. Low ROI

Although, the growth in this segment of animal health is huge with a high potential for future expansions and new entries, the current market size and vaccine volumes are not high enough to set-up the production plant with high capital investment in the country. The lack of ROI is a deterrent for new players to enter the industry.

3. Lack of Trained Personnel

Also there is a dearth of trained personal and veterinarians to cater to the growing but scattered pet population.

4.4 Change in Numbers of Veterinary Institution in different States of India in Recent Time

Department of Animal Husbandry Dairying and Fisheries publish annually the report of the department work. From these recent reports here we tried to show

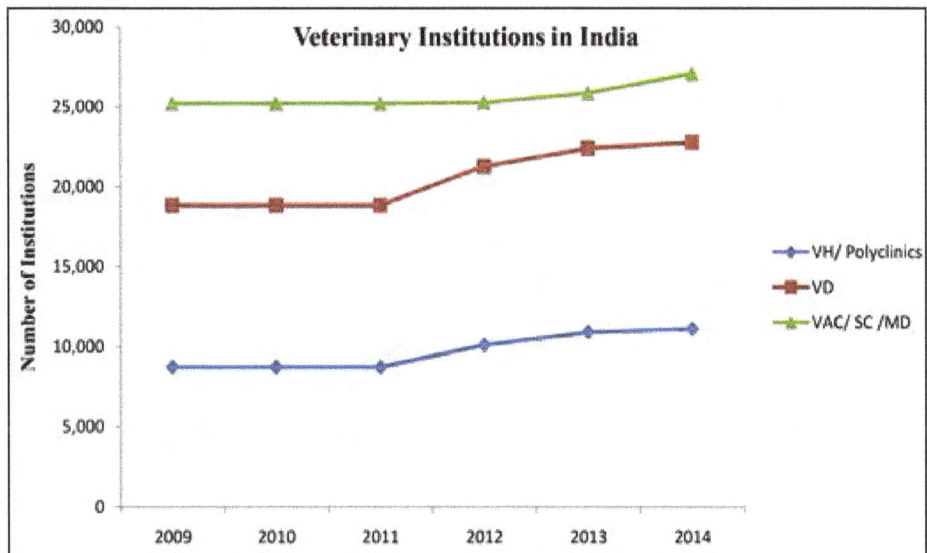

Figure 4.17: Growth of Veterinary Institution in India in Last Five Years (2009-2014).
VAC/SC/MD: Veterinary Aid Centre/Stockmen Centre/Mobile Dispensaries; VD: Veterinary Dispensaries; VH/Polyclinics: Veterinary Hospitals/Polyclinics.

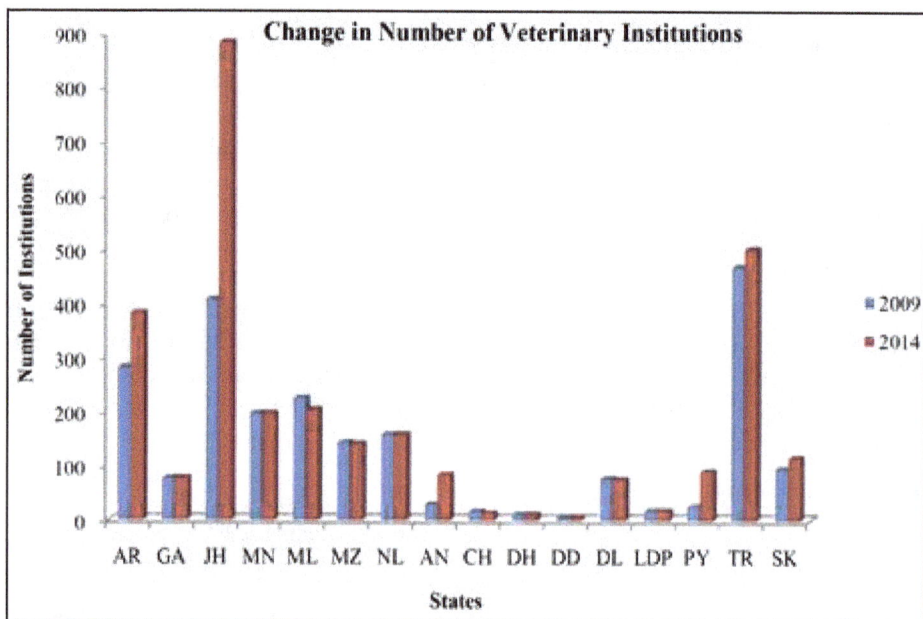

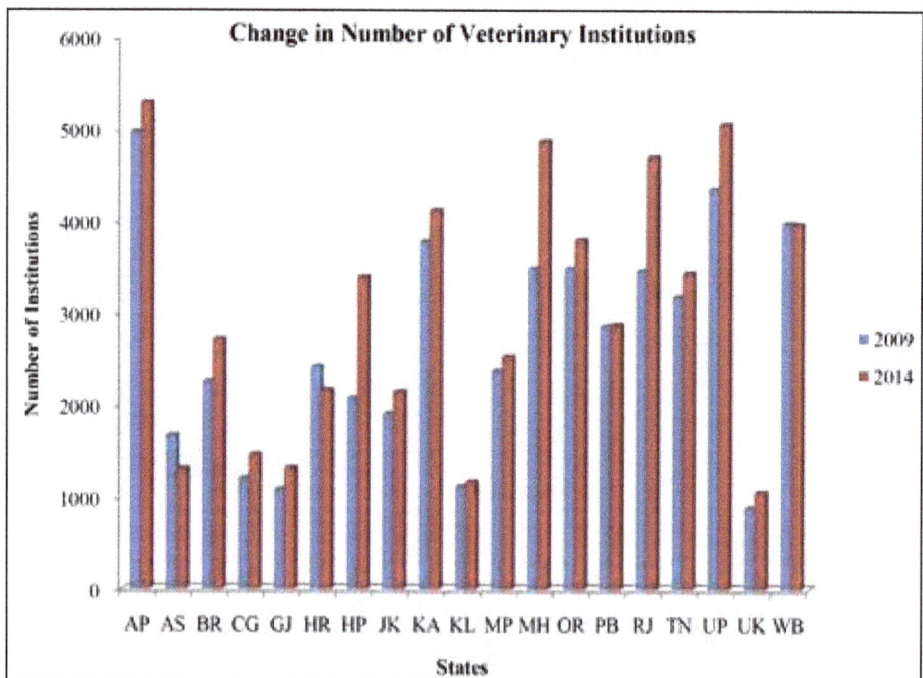

Figure 4.10: State wise Growth Veterinary Institution during Last Five Years (2009-2014).

the trend of change in numbers of veterinary institutes in different states of India (Figures 4.17 and 4.18).

4.5 Predicted Population of Animals in India in 2032

The prediction of animal population in this section is done based on the Compound Annual Growth Rate (CAGR) from 2012 to 2032 as shown in Figure 4.19A-D.

4.6 Private Vet Clinics and Pet Shops

In the present day, most veterinary clinics are found together with pet shops catering to the various requirements of the pets. Various pet accessories and animal supplies are available in pet shop which includes food cages, treats, toys, collars, leashes, cat litter and aquariums.

4.6.1 Framework for Governing Legal Pet Shops

The Animal Welfare Board in India reported a draft regarding the **Pet Shops Rules, 2010** developed by honour of ability conferred by section 38 of the Prevention of Cruelty to Animals Act, 1960 which was published by Ministry of Environment, Forest and Climate Change, GoI. To know the details regarding the terms and conditions for licensing of pet shops refer the reference note.

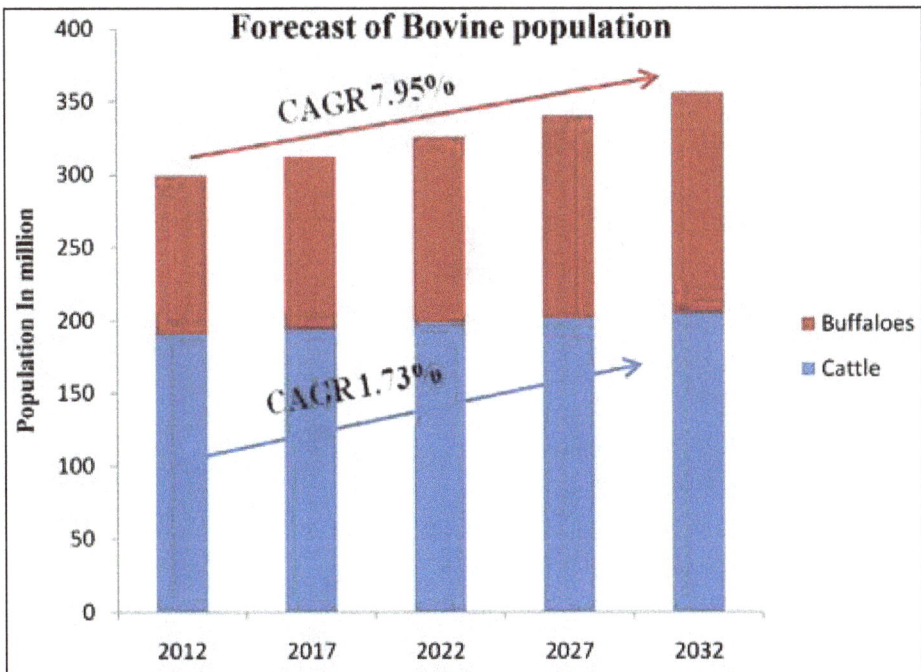

Figure 4.19A: Animal Population Forecast in India (2012-2032) (Based on CAGR).

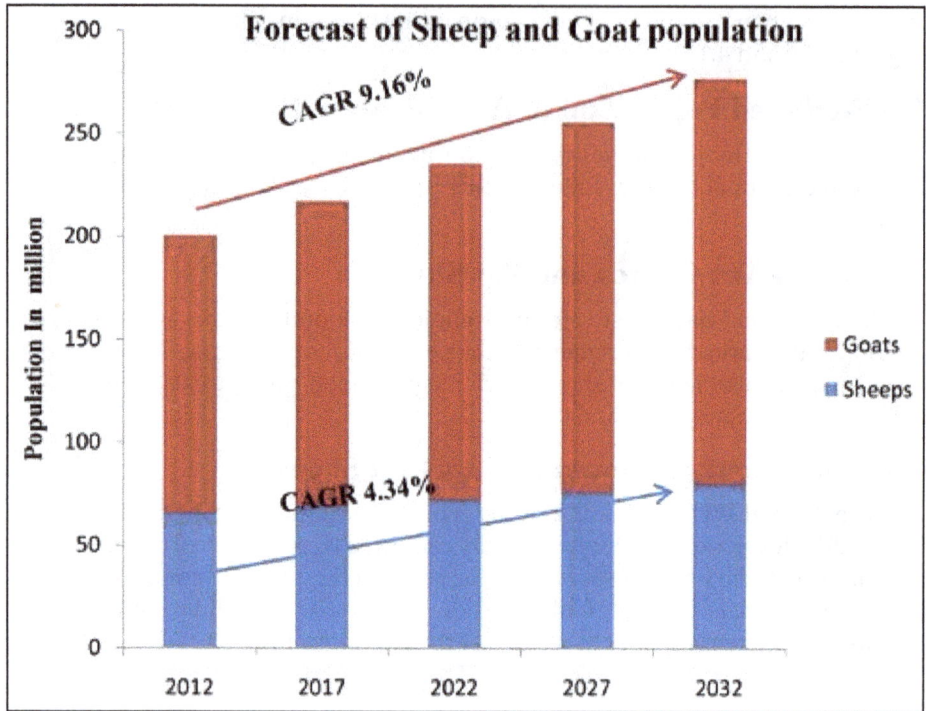

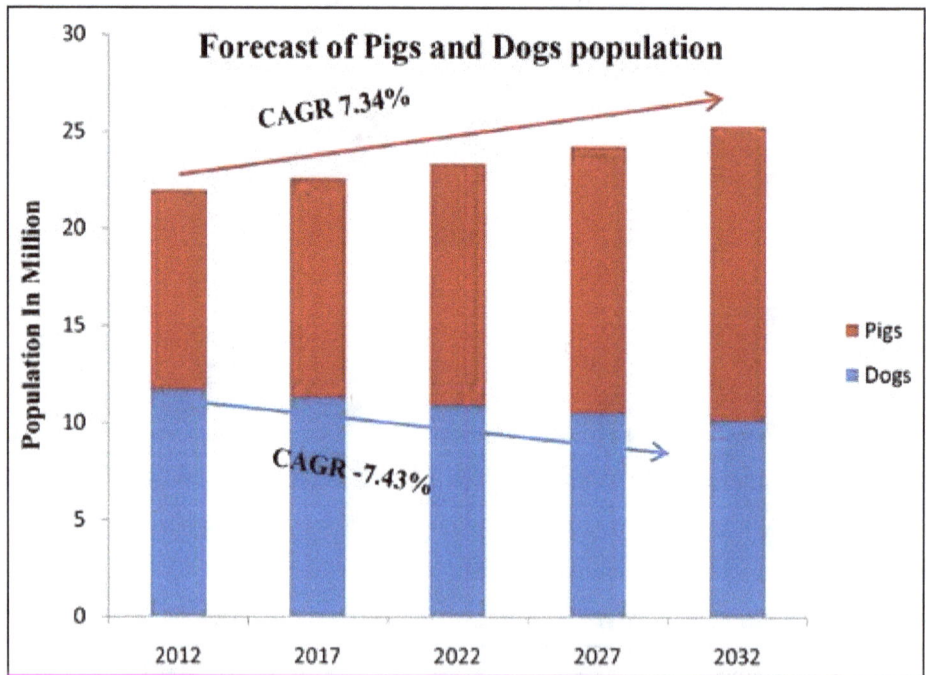

Figure 4.19B: Animal Population Forecast in India (2012-2032) (Based on CAGR).

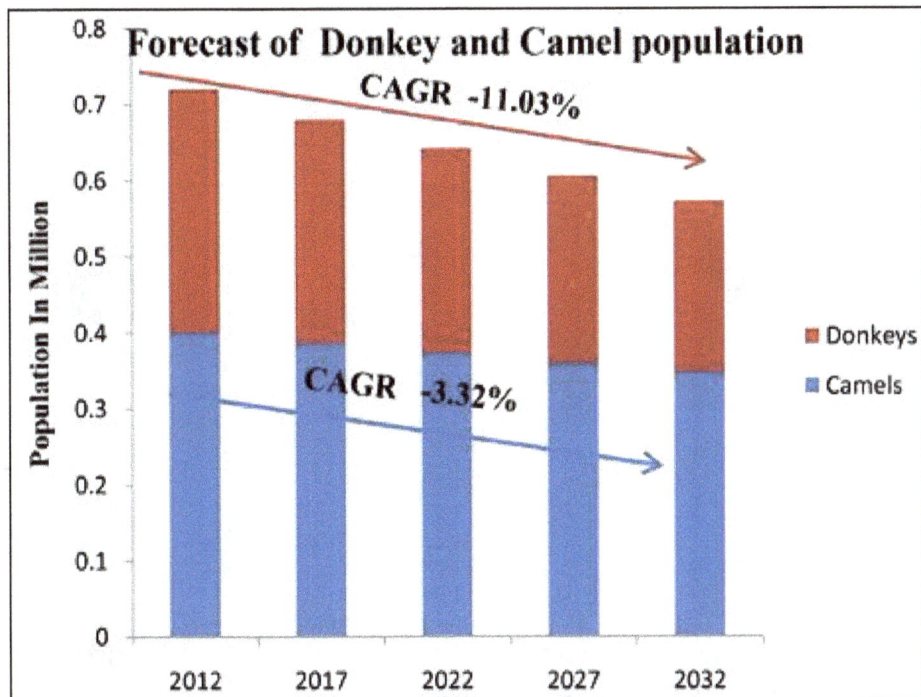

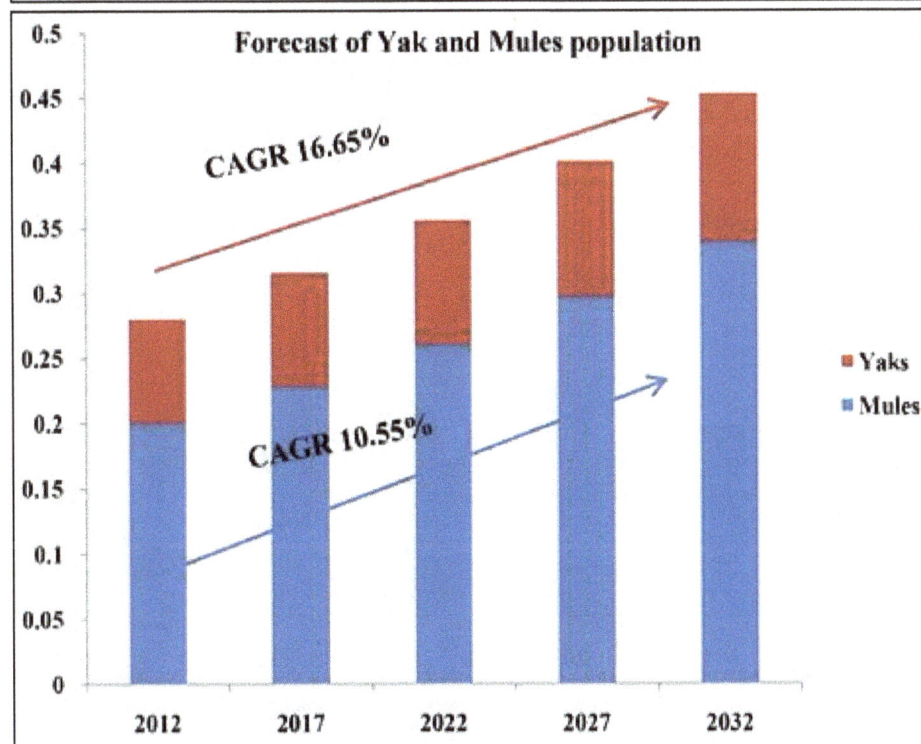

Figure 4.19C: Animal Population Forecast in India (2012-2032) (Based on CAGR).

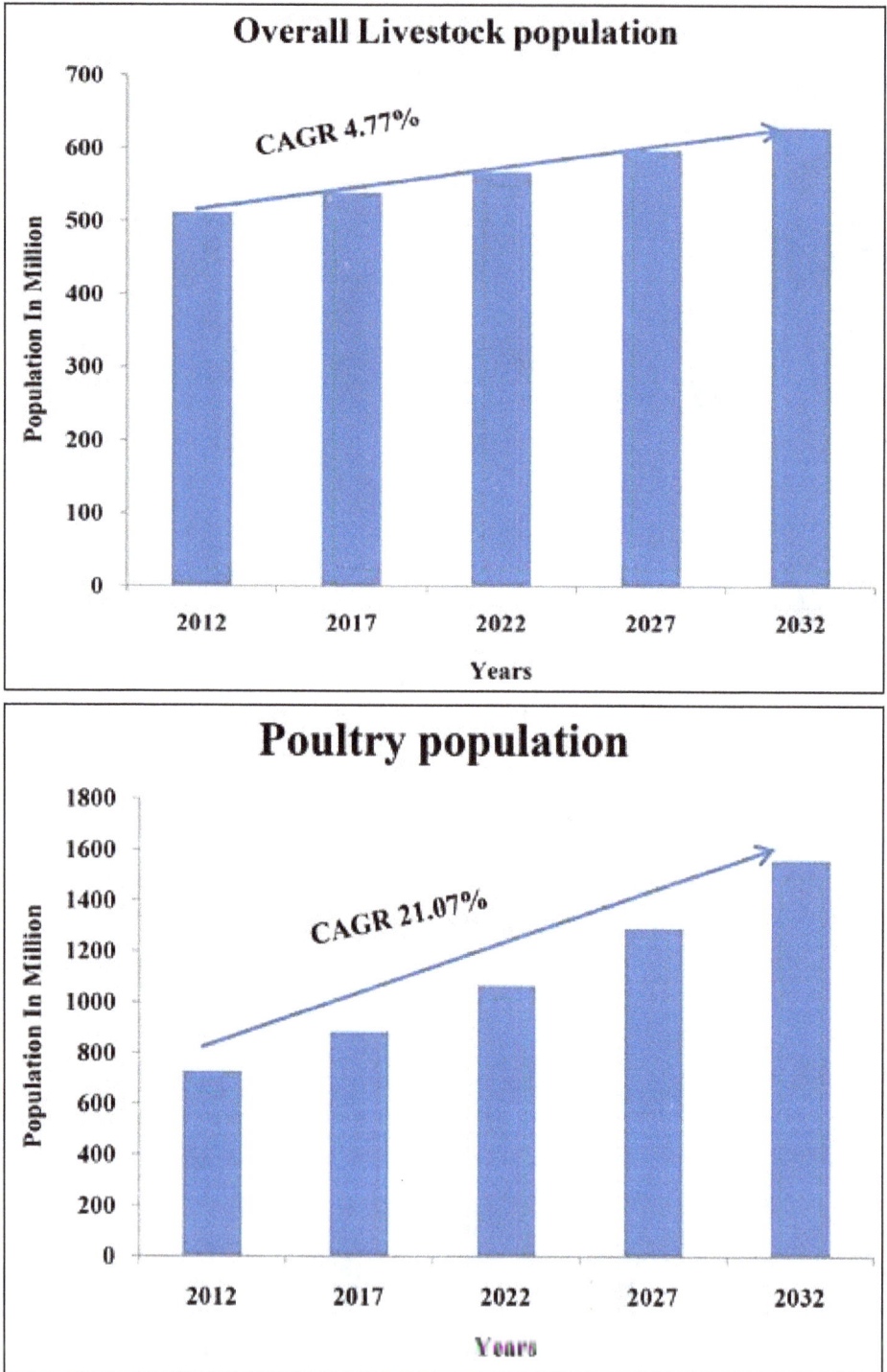

Figure 4.19D: Animal Population Forecast in India (2012-2032) (Based on CAGR).

4.6.2 Application to Local Authority for Establishing License

SCHEDULE I

To

The Local Authority (As defined in the Rules)

Copy to:

Animal Welfare Board of India Subject : Application for grant of license for Pet Shop Sir,

I/We _____, r/o/with office address _____, do hereby apply for a license to operate/continue operating a Pet Shop at _____ in accordance with the particulars set out below:

1. Name and address of the pet shop premises:

2. Full name and address of proposed pet shop owner:

3. Telephone number:

4. Details of accommodation/infrastructure available at proposed pet shop premises :

5. Working hours and rest day, *i.e.* day on which shop shall remain closed:

6. Ventilation arrangement:

7. Lighting arrangement:

8. Heating/cooling arrangement, and how comfortable temperature will be maintained :

9. Arrangements for food storage:

10. Cleanliness, how proposed to be maintained, and arrangements for removal of animal excreta :

11. Arrangement for disposal of animals that die:

12. Arrangement for provision of medical and veterinary attention:

13. Details of pet animals proposed to be displayed or house in the Pet Shop for sale:

TYPES OF ANIMALS:

NUMBER OF EACH TYPE OF ANIMAL:

AGE/S OF EACH TYPE OF ANIMAL:

ACCOMODATION/NUMBER AND SIZE OF CAGES/ENCLOSURES:

14. Details of cheque/demand draft number for payment of fee:

I/We do hereby declare that the information provided by us is accurate and true.

Place: Signature of Applicant

Date:

4.6.3 Status of Pet Shops in Chennai

A small study was undertaken to assess the status of pet shops in Chennai city.

Various feed types, huge number of cosmetic products and accessories are sold in these shops. About 21 types of breeds exist in Chennai. Almost all regions in Chennai were found accessible with pet clinics and shops as depicted in Figure 4.20.

   ✰ **North Chennai region – (**Tiruvottiyur, Manali, Madhavaram, Tondiarpet and Royapuram, Basin Bridge)

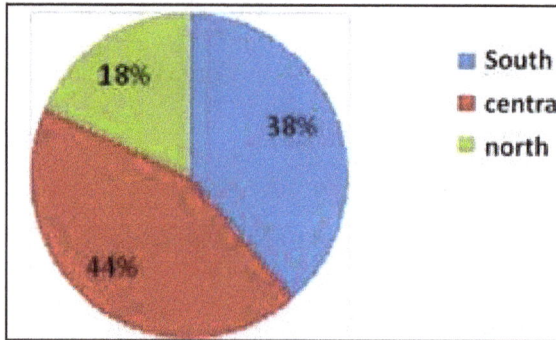

Figure 4.20: Pet Shop Status Region-wise Chennai.

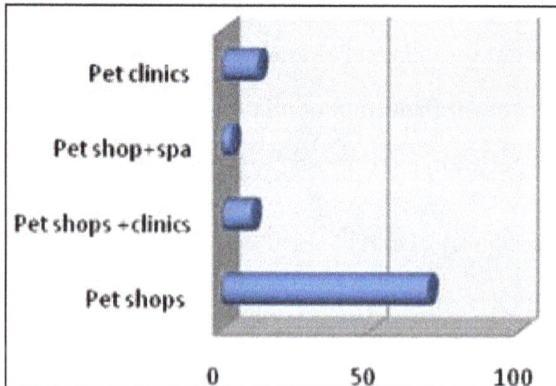

Figure 4.21: List of Pet Clinics and Shops in Chennai.

☆ **Central Chennai region** – (Thiru-Vi-Ka Nagar, Ambattur, Anna Nagar, Teynampet and Kodambakkam, Shenoy Nagar) and

☆ **South Chennai region** – (Valasaravakkam, Alandur, Adyar, Perungudi, Sholinganallur and Saidapet)

There were about 34 pet shops, 39 pet clinics and 7 kennel club/training centres in Chennai as shown in Figure 4.21 and list of items sold in Chennai pet shops in Figure 4.22.

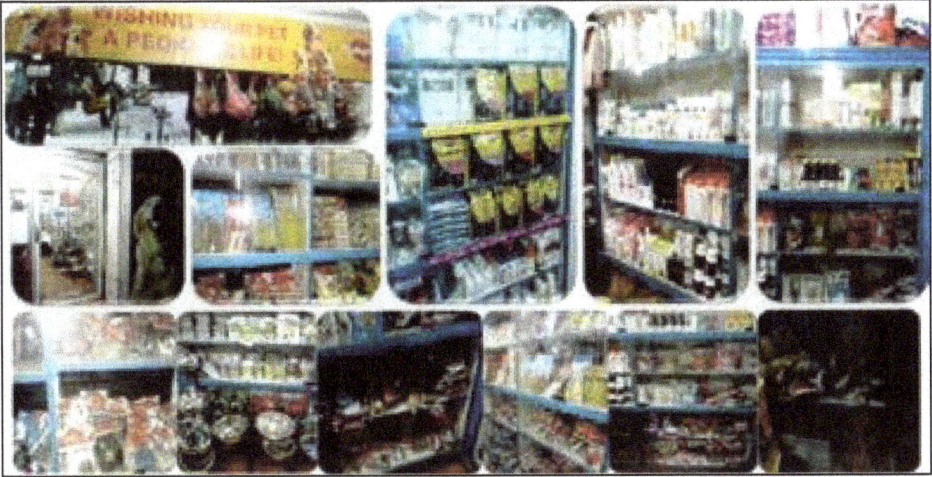

Figure 4. 22: Items for Sale in Pet Shops at Chennai.

Reference

Report No.261, Need to Regulate Pet shops and Dog and Aquarium Fish Breeding-2015, Law Commission of India, Govt of India.

5

Economic Impact of Diseases

5.1 Introduction

There are many animal diseases that causes an irreparable economic loss to the farming community. These diseases can affect all types of animals like poultry, dairy and food animals. The economically important bovine diseases are FMD, Brucellosis, mastitis, Surra, Haemorrhagic Septicaemia *etc.* In small ruminants FMD, Pox, Anthrax, PPR and Enterotoxemia are the main economically important diseases. In poultry economically important diseases are ND, Marek's disease and IBD. In this chapter information available on the economic impact of a few animal diseases is given.

5.2 Bovine Diseases

The economic losses due to bovine diseases are shown in Figure 5.1.

a) **Mastitis** condition is reported to cause an economic loss of Rs. 1248.67/ animal - Singh *et al.* (2014) *Veterinary World* 7.8: 579-585.

b) **Surra** disease is reported to cause loss of Rs. 6824.4/animal - Singh *et al.* (2014) *Veterinary World* 7.8: 579-585.

c) **Haemorrhagic Septicaemia (cattle)** disease is reported to cause an annual economic loss of Rs. 6816/animal in India - Singh *et al.* (2014) *Agricultural Economics Research Review* 27.2: 271-279.

d) **Haemorrhagic Septicaemia (buffalo)** disease is reported to cause an annual economic loss of Rs. 10901/animal in India - Singh *et al.* (2014) *Agricultural Economics Research Review* 27.2: 271-279.

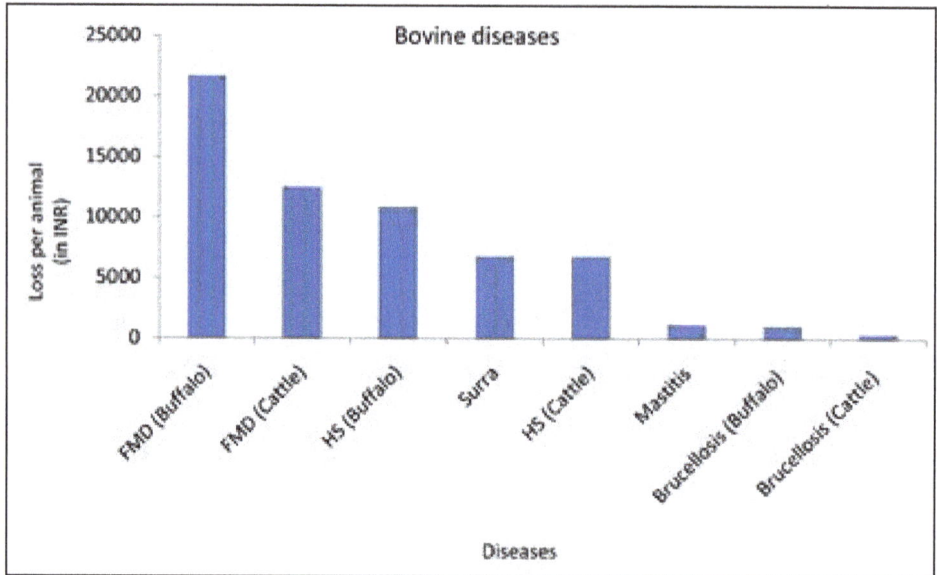

Figure 5.1: Economic Loss due to Bovine Diseases.

e) **Brucellosis (cattle)** disease is reported to cause per animal economic loss of 6.8 US Dollars (Rs. 408) - Singh *et al.* (2015) *Preventive Veterinary Medicine* 119.3: 211-215

f) **Brucellosis (buffalo)** disease is reported to cause per animal economic loss of 18.2 US Dollars (Rs. 1092) - Singh *et al.* (2015) *Preventive Veterinary Medicine* 119.3: 211-215

g) **Foot and Mouth disease (cattle)** is reported to cause per animal economic loss of Rs. 12,532 (Singh *et al.* (2013) *The Indian Journal of Animal Sciences* 83.9: 964–970

h) **Foot and Mouth disease (buffalo)** is reported to cause per animal economic loss of Rs. 21,682 (Singh *et al.* (2013) *The Indian Journal of Animal Sciences* 83.9:964–970

5.3 Caprine and Ovine Diseases

Economic losses due to Caprine and Ovine Diseases are shown in Figure 5.2.

a) **Foot and mouth disease** is reported to cause economic loss of Rs. 37.80 lakhs/annum in India - Singh and Prasad (2008) *Agricultural Economics Research Review* 21.2: 297-302

b) **Anthrax** disease is reported to cause economic loss of Rs. 5.17 lakhs/annum in India - Singh and Prasad (2008) *Agricultural Economics Research Review* 21.2: 297-302

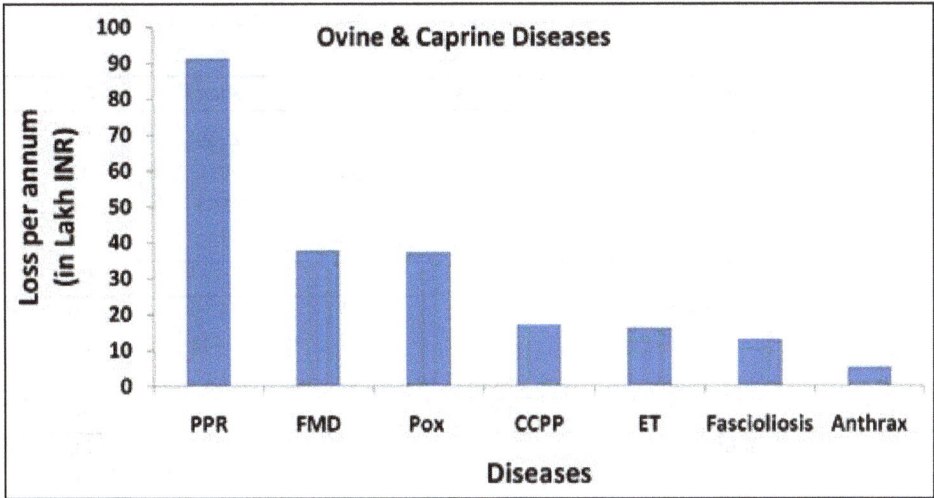

Figure 5.2: Economic Loss due to Caprine and Ovine Diseases.

c) **Sheep and goat pox** disease is reported to cause economic loss of Rs. 37.25 lakhs/annum in India - Singh and Prasad (2008) *Agricultural Economics Research Review* 21.2: 297-302

d) **Fascioliasis/Distomatosis** disease is reported to cause economic loss of Rs. 13.12 lakhs/annum in India - Singh and Prasad (2008) *Agricultural Economics Research Review* 21.2: 297-302

c) **Enterotoxemia** disease is reported to cause economic loss of Rs. 16.18 lakhs/annum in India - Singh and Prasad (2008) *Agricultural Economics Research Review* 21.2: 297-302

d) **Peste des Petits Ruminants (PPR)** disease is reported to cause economic loss of Rs. 91.42 lakhs/annum in India - Singh and Prasad (2008) *Agricultural Economics Research Review* 21.2: 297-302.

e) **Contagious caprine pleuropneumonia** disease is reported to cause economic loss of Rs. 17.04 lakhs/annum in India - Singh and Prasad (2008) *Agricultural Economics Research Review*21.2: 297-302.

f) *Brucella melitensis* **(sheep)** disease is reported to cause economic loss of Rs. 1180/animal in India - Sulima and Venkataraman (2010) *Tamil Nadu Journal of Veterinary and Animal Sciences* 6: 191-192.

g) *Brucella melitensis* **(goats)** disease is reported to cause economic loss of Rs. 2121.82/animal) in India - Sulima and Venkataraman (2010) *Tamil Nadu Journal of Veterinary and Animal Sciences* 6: 191-192.

5.4 Porcine Diseases

a) **Brucellosis** disease is reported to cause annual economic loss of 0.6 US Dollars/Rs. 36 (1 US $ = Rs. 60/-) per animal in India - Singh *et al.* (2015) *Preventive Veterinary Medicine* 119.3: 211-215

Animal Biotechnology: Vaccines and Diagnostics

**Table 5.1: Species-wise Incidence of Livestock Disease in India
during January-December, 2014**

Sl.No.	Disease	Species	Outbreak	Attack	Death
1.	Foot and Mouth Disease	Bov	168	20595	1582
		Buff	33	4638	127
		O/C	26	794	86
		Swi	11	189	27
		Total	238	26216	1822
2.	Heamorrhagic septiceamia	Bov	93	3219	304
		Buff	32	3444	201
		O/C	6	153	36
		Total	131	6816	541
3.	Black Quarter	Bov	114	4263	288
		Buff	4	22	9
		Total	118	4285	297
4.	Anthrax	Bov	30	1878	1878
		O/C	25	302	302
		Total	55	2180	2180
5.	Fascioliasis	Bov	129	3606	4
		O/C	43	1701	48
		Buff	17	688	0
		Avian	1	10	0
		Swine	2	4	0
		Total	192	6009	52
6.	Enterotoxemia	O/C	44	1374	308
		Bov	4	12	0
		Buff	2	2	0
		Total	50	1388	308
7.	Sheep and Goat Pox	O/C	77	2420	472
		Bov	4	69	12
		Avian	6	155	19
		Canine	1	6	0
		Total	88	2650	503
8.	Blue Tongue	O/C	14	659	145
	C.C.P.P.	O/C	2	29	5
	Amphistomiasis	Bov	104	14225	26
		O/C	39	2301	0
		Buff	11	234	0
		Total	154	16760	26
9.	Schistosomiasis	Bov	49	900	0
		Buff	52	7	35
		Total	101	907	35

b) **Cystic echinococcosis** disease is reported to cause economic loss of Rs. 961,41,417/annum in India - Singh *et al.* (2014) *Preventive Veterinary Medicine* 113.1: 1-12.

5.5 Poultry diseases

a) **Infectious bursal disease (IBD)** was reported to cause economic loss of Rs. 11149 per 1000 birds - S. Selvam (2000), M. V. Sc. Thesis, *Madras Veterinary College Chennai.*

b) **Ranikhet disease** disease reported to cause economic loss of Rs. 6845 per 1000 birds - S. Selvam (2000), M. V. Sc. Thesis, *Madras Veterinary College Chennai.*

5.6 Loss of Government's wealth

For livestock health government is helping farmers by implementing different disease control programs. In these programs extensive vaccination of animals is going on in different parts of India. Rs 3,114 crore have been allocated for the Livestock Health and Disease Control Programmes in the Twelfth Five Year Plan. Some of the main programmes are:

☆ Foot and Mouth Disease Control Programme (FMD-CP)

☆ National Animal Disease Reporting System (NADRS)

☆ Peste des Petits Ruminants Control Programme (PPR-CP)

☆ Brucellosis Control Programme (Brucellosis - CP)

☆ Establishment and Strengthening of existing Veterinary Hospitals and Dispensaries (ESVHD)

☆ Classical Swine Fever Control Programme (CSF-CP)

☆ Avian Influenza: Preparedness, Control and Containment

Compensation Money

From 2006 -2015 there were 24 outbreaks of avian influenza reported. For this Government has given the compensation of Rs. 2,429.92 lakhs to farmers.

6

Vaccines

6.1 Introduction

Louis Pasteur first used the term vaccine in 1881 and demonstrated the feasibility of inactivating or attenuating microbes. Studies with fowl cholera and anthrax led to the concepts of inactivation as a means to reduce the virulence of microorganisms. Serial passage of erysipelas and rabies organisms in animals (primarily rabbits or lapinization) demonstrated attenuation as an alternative strategy to reduce or eliminate virulence.

These developments eventually led to successful immunization programs against typhoid fever, tuberculosis, rinderpest and foot and mouth disease (FMD).

As technical advances were embraced by the vaccine industry, regulations and guidelines for registration of new biologicals as well as consistent manufacture of pure, safe and potent vaccines were established. These regulations ensured consistent potency, safety and purity of vaccines. Good manufacturing practices guidelines and master seed and master cell stock requirements have further ensured consistent manufacture of vaccines that will provide consistent immunogenicity and efficacy. A veterinarian therefore may use with confidence any approved vaccine as recommended by the manufacturer to achieve the anticipated clinical outcome of protection.

Properties of Ideal Vaccine

☆ Safe in young ones and immune compromised hosts

☆ Provide long lasting protective immunity.

☆ Induce humoral, mucosal and cellular immunity.

☆ Not to induce autoimmunity or hypersensitivity.

☆ Inexpensive to produce, easy to store, transport and administer.

The vaccine vial may contain relevant antigen, adjuvant (usually alum), preservatives and/or traces of protein derived from the cells in which the vaccine agent was cultured *e.g.* egg protein.

The vaccine development and production is generally dependent upon

☆ Severity of the disease

☆ Economic impact

☆ Availability of safe and potent vaccine to combat infection

☆ Vaccine production parameters to assess safety and efficiency

In India in the last 10 years only two new vaccines have been developed and introduced

☆ Peste des petits ruminants – live attenuated vaccine by IVRI

☆ Bluetongue vaccine with 5 serotypes – Inactivated vaccine by ICAR/TANUVAS

☆ Johne's disease vaccine - inactivated vaccine by CSIR

6.2 Types of Vaccine

The various types of vaccines are:

☆ Live, attenuated vaccines

☆ Inactivated vaccines

☆ Subunit vaccines

☆ DNA vaccines

☆ Recombinant vector vaccines

6.2.1 Live Attenuated Vaccine

☆ This uses a non-pathogenic form of the infectious organism, limited in its ability to replicate in the host and therefore unable to cause disease.

☆ An attenuated microbe simulates an infection without causing disease pathology.

☆ Attenuation done by growing microbe in abnormal conditions like low temperature/heterologous hosts. Because it has adapted to grow in extreme conditions, it has limited growth in normal environment or by modifying genes needed for replication – site directed mutagenesis.

Advantages

☆ Broad humoral and CTL responses.

☆ Attenuated organism replicates within the host and induces memory.

☆ Most vaccines require one exposure.

☆ Vaccine can be administered at the normal route of entry, ensuring protection at this site.

☆ Vaccines elicit mucosal immune responses.

Disadvantages

☆ Danger of reversion of attenuated form to virulent form.

☆ Attenuated strain could recombine with natural pathogenic strain resulting in new form.

☆ Difficult to prepare.

☆ Growth culture could be contaminated with other substances.

6.2.2 Inactivated Vaccine

Inactivated vaccines are made by killing or inactivating a pathogen by heat, or chemical means. The inactivation ensures that the pathogen can no longer replicate within the host but would generate immune responses.

Advantages

☆ Uses pathogen that is killed and no longer capable of replicating within the host.

☆ It is easily phagocytosed and presented to T_h cells.

☆ The full range of antigens is presented ensuring a broad immune response.

☆ Since the organism is dead – no disease in host.

☆ Vaccine is relatively heat stable.

Disadvantages

☆ Inactivated vaccines produce a strong humoral response but weak CTL mediated response.

☆ No replication in host – presence of antigen is short-lived – requires booster vaccinations.

☆ Many pathogens have endotoxins that are not removed – cause serious side effects.

☆ Inadequate killing cause disease.

6.2.3 Subunit Vaccines

☆ DNA coding for an immunogenic protein of a pathogen can be inserted into either bacteria, yeast, viruses which infect mammalian cells or by transfection of mammalian cells. The cells will then produce the protein endogenously and the protein can be harvested.

☆ Large amounts of antigen can be produced inexpensively.

☆ Genetic manipulation of antigen possible. Antigens can be made more immunogenic or can be genetically inactivated.

Advantages

☆ Safe to use on immuno suppressed individuals.

☆ Less possibility of side effects.

Disadvantages

☆ Immune responses are primarily humoral. The antigens are processed via the MHC class II pathway and therefore do not induce CTL response.

☆ For example, the gene coding for the surface protein of hepatitis B virus is over expressed in yeast. Antigen self assembles forming aggregates resembling viral particles which are then secreted and purified.

6.2.4 DNA Vaccines

☆ Genes encoding antigens of an infectious organism are expressed by the host's own cells.

☆ Genes are inserted into a bacterial plasmid under the control of a mammalian promoter. The chimeric plasmid is directly injected into muscle or the DNA is absorbed to a solid matrix such as gold particles and injected intracutaneously by a gene gun. These particles are taken up by skin cells and the genes are expressed as in a viral vector.

Advantages

☆ Full spectrum of immune responses:

  ❑ Safety

  ❑ No risk of disease as in live attenuated vaccines

  ❑ No injection site reactions as in subunit vaccines given with adjuvant.

☆ Neonates can be vaccinated with minimal interference with passive maternal antibody.

☆ Can be used in immuno-compromised animals (since there is no replicating pathogen).

☆ Thermostable.

☆ Low cost production and administration.

☆ Multicomponent vaccine in a single dose.

☆ Marker vaccines – differentiate vaccinates from infected.

Disadvantages

☆ Slow rising antibody titre.

☆ Potential for integration of DNA into host genome.

☆ Development of auto immunity.

6.2.5 Recombinant Vector Vaccine

☆ Genes encoding antigens of pathogenic organisms are inserted into attenuated live vectors. The recombinant virus/bacteria are then able to replicate in and display the inserted proteins to the host.

☆ Both class I and II MHC pathway presentation.

☆ Can be targeted by viral tropisms for particular cells.

Advantages

☆ These vectors are easy to grow and are basically safe.

☆ Multi component vaccines possible.

Disadvantages

☆ The live virus vector being used does have the risk of reversion to virulence.

☆ Some vectors such as Adenovirus can transform cells into a cancerous phenotype. Even if oncogenes are removed, vector virus can recombine with naturally occurring pathogenic strains in the environment and form a new hybrid virus with transforming properties. Examples are Vaccinia, Canary pox, Avipox, Adeno, Herpes viruses.

☆ Induction of antibodies against vectors has the potential to neutralize subsequent doses of the vaccine.

Some of the recombinant veterinary vaccines presently in clinical trials and development include

☆ Porcine Corona virus in pigs

☆ Pseudorabies virus in pigs

☆ Classical swine fever virus in pigs

☆ Bovine herpes virus-1 in cattle

☆ Equine influenza virus in horses

☆ West Nile virus in horses

☆ MDV (HVT) and IBDV in poultry

☆ Newcastle disease virus in poultry

☆ Avian influenza virus in poultry

☆ Rabies virus for cats, canines and wildlife

☆ Feline leukemia virus in cats

☆ Canine parvovirus 1 in dogs

☆ Canine corona virus in dogs

☆ Canine distemper virus in dogs

Table 6.1: Comparison Features of Various Vaccines

Feature	Attenuated	Inactivated	Live Recombinant	Protein Vaccine	Peptide Vaccine	DNA Vaccine
Antibody response	+	+	+	+	+	+
Antibody rise	Fast	Fast	Fast	Fast	Fast	Slow
CTL induction	Yes	No	Yes	No	Variable	Yes
T-helper induction	+	+	+	+	+	+
Complete antigen repertoire	Yes	Yes	No	No	No	Possible
IR to vaccine carrier	–	–	Possible	–	–	–
Duration of response	Long	Short	Long	Short	Short	Long
No. of required vaccine dose	One	Multiple	Multiple	Multiple	Multiple	One or more
Safety	No	Yes	No	Yes	Yes	Probably
Risk of reversion	Yes	No	Yes	No	No	No
Efficacy in the presence of maternal antibodies	Yes	Yes	Yes	Yes	Yes	No
Ease of production	Variable	Difficult	Difficult	Difficult	Difficult	Easy
Cost	Variable	Expensive	Expensive	Expensive	Expensive	Inexpensive

With respect to recombinant veterinary vaccines only a few have been licensed globally. Two veterinary DNA vaccines have so far been granted regulatory approvals. The US FDA has granted a license to Fort Dodge, a subsidiary of Wyeth, to market West Nile Innovator DNA, a vaccine to prevent West Nile virus infection in horses. Also, the Canadian Food Inspection Agency (CFIA) has granted license to Aqua Health Limited, a subsidiary of Novartis, to market APEX-IHN, a DNA vaccine to protect farm-raised salmon fish against infectious haematopoietic necrosis virus. So far, no DNA vaccine has been licensed for use in humans.

6.3 Veterinary Vaccines

Animal and Poultry vaccines rely largely on exotic vaccine candidates isolated elsewhere in the world more than 50 – 60 years ago

Disease	Strains	Year of Isolation	Details
New Castle Disease	Lasota strain	1946	Farm Adam LaSota, New Jersey
	Komarov	1946	Komarov and Goldsmith, 1946
	Mukteswar	1945 (introduced)	India
	Fuller		India
Marek's Disease	HVT	1970	Marek, Hungary
Infectious Bursal Disease	Lukert strain	1962	Gumboro, Delaware
Infectious Bronchitis	Massachusetts	1940	USA
Infectious Laryngeal	A20	1950	Australia
Tracheitis	SA2	1950	Australia
	Strain w93	1950s	China
Canine Distemper virus	Onderstepoort	1923	Puntoni, Italy (isolated)
Canine Parvo virus	Cornell strain	1989	USA

6.4 Company profiles

Indovax

Indovax Private Limited is a principal maker of biologics in India since 1986. The company is one of the leaders in development, manufacture and marketing of poultry vaccines. The company has an assessed overall national market share of over twenty five per cent and produces over four billion doses of vaccine annually that provide to the needs of the domestic and international markets. This leadership is maintained by a team of competent scientists drawn from various disciplines that include virology, microbiology, immunology, biotechnology, pathology and epidemiology. The services are located at Hisar. It has independent production facilities, quality control laboratories, animal testing facilities and a Science and Technology center (*http://www.indovax.com*).

Brilliant Biopharma

BBPPL was established up in 1998 at Hyderabad to manufacture and market Veterinary Biologicals and Medicines. The Company produces several viral and bacterial vaccines. All the primary batches of vaccines were tested and certified by Indian Veterinary Research Institute (IVRI). The manufacturing capacity is attributed with WHO-GMP and ISO 9001-2008 certifications as well as Good Laboratory Practices (GLP) certificate. The company has its credit the awards like 'National Award for Safety', 'National Award for Environment' and the 'National Award for R&D' (*http://brilliantbiopharma.com*).

Hester Biosciences

Hester Biosciences Limited is a WHO-GMP, ISO 9001:2008, ISO 14001:2004, OHSAS18001:2007 and GLP certified company, developing animal vaccines and health products. It is situated near the city of Ahmedabad, Gujarat, Western India. Product range contains vaccines, health products and diagnostics. The services include seroprofiling for poultry flocks and mastitis control plans for cattle (*http://www.hester.in*).

Indian Immunologicals (IIL)

Indian Immunologicals Ltd. (IIL) was setup by the National Dairy Development Board (NDDB) in 1982 with the objective of making Foot and Mouth Disease (FMD) vaccine available to farmers at a reasonable price. The technology for FMD vaccine manufacture was acquired from M/s. Wellcome Foundation Limited, United Kingdom (*http://www.indimmune.com*).

The plant in Hyderabad currently has a capacity of 250 million trivalent doses of FMD vaccine. IIL launched the tissue culture vaccine "Raksharab" in 1989. It functions as one of the largest plants in the world for veterinary vaccines which is WHO-GMP and ISO-9001 certified. IIL caters to the mandate of NDDB to deliver products and facilities to improve the value of livestock in the country. IIL is the second company in the world and first in India to launch the purified Vero cell rabies vaccine (PVRV).

Intervet

MSD-Animal health is a worldwide, research-driven concern that produces and markets a broad range of veterinary medicines and services. They are extremely active, robust and diversified company with a robust, scientifically-proven, product range and an ever-growing global extent. The products have been marketed over 140 countries and have one of the best research and development (R&D) facilities around the world (*http://www.msd-animal-health.co.in*).

Bio-Med

Bio-Med (P) Limited boarded on its principled mission of producing world-class vaccines vital to the needs of a developing country. The company was listed and combined for the manufacture of vaccines to protect animals and humans against infectious diseases. Bio-Med got the Drug Manufacturing license from the State Government for manufacturing Poultry Vaccines in December 1974 and developed the first poultry vaccine manufacturing element of the private sector in the state (*http://www.biomed.co.in*).

6.5 Veterinary Vaccines Available in India

There are different kinds of veterinary vaccines available in India. These can be differentiated by species and choice of immunogen and can further be divided as live, inactivated and recombinant.

Various types of microbial vaccine and species-wise vaccines availability were given in Figure 6.1 in percentage. Figures 6.2–6.4 represents types of vaccines produced and various types of bacterial and viral vaccines available in India.

Diseases

Bio-Med

* ☆ Indian vaccine manufacturers produce more poultry vaccine than livestock and companion vaccines
* ☆ All of the State biologicals manufacture HS and BQ vaccines.
* ☆ Most viral vaccines are produced against
* ☆ NDV (8)
* ☆ IBD (8)
* ☆ Rabies (7)
* ☆ Fowl Pox (6) and IBV (6)

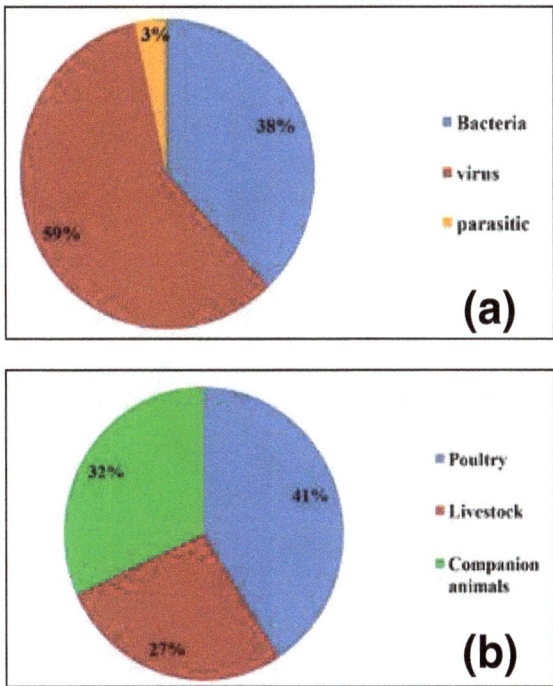

Figure 6.1: Types of Vaccine Available.
(a) Microbial Vaccine; (b) Species-wise Vaccine.

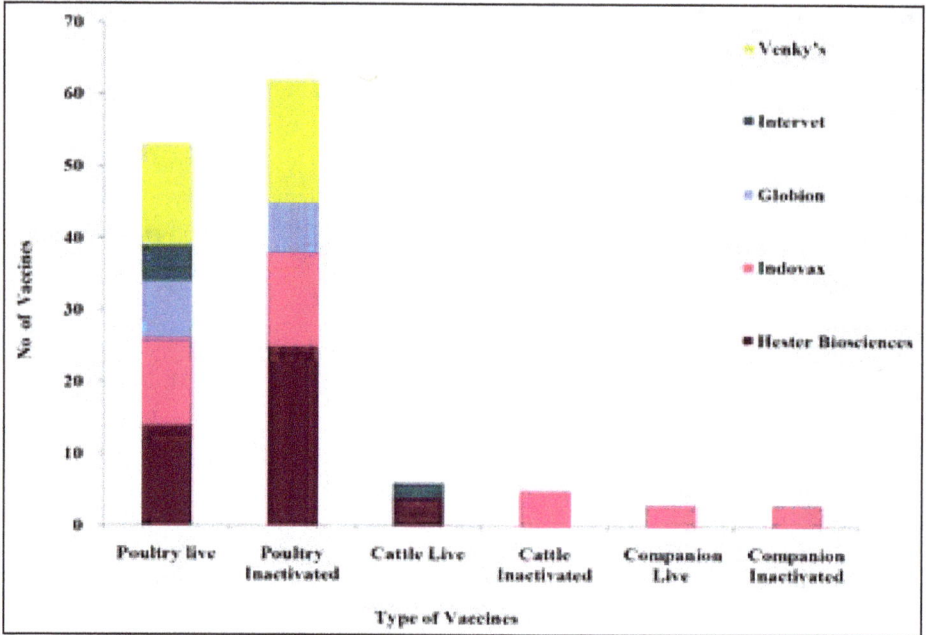

Figure 6.2: Species-wise Vaccine Availability in Various Company Product Range.

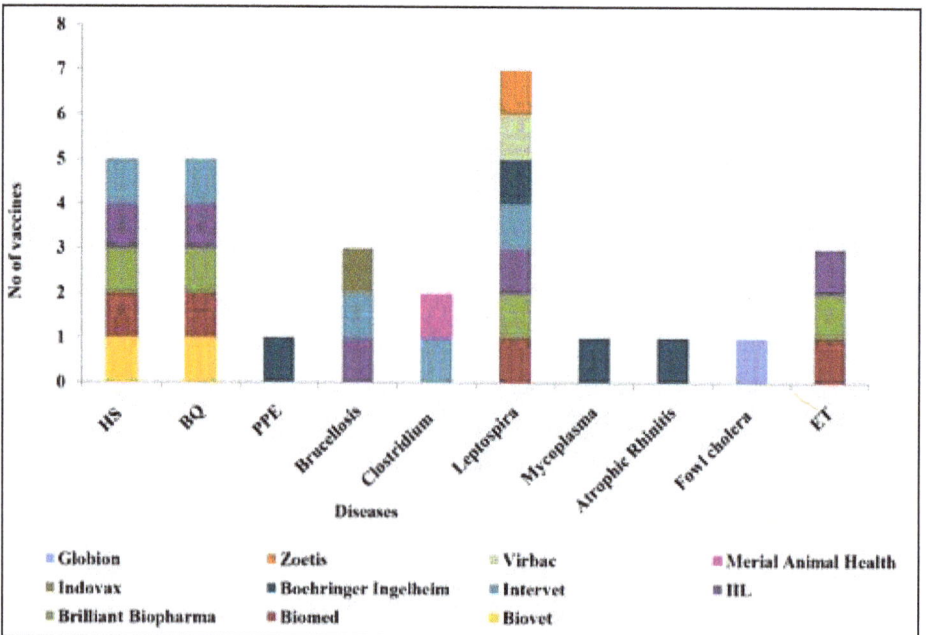

Figure 6.3: Types of Bacterial Vaccines Available in India.

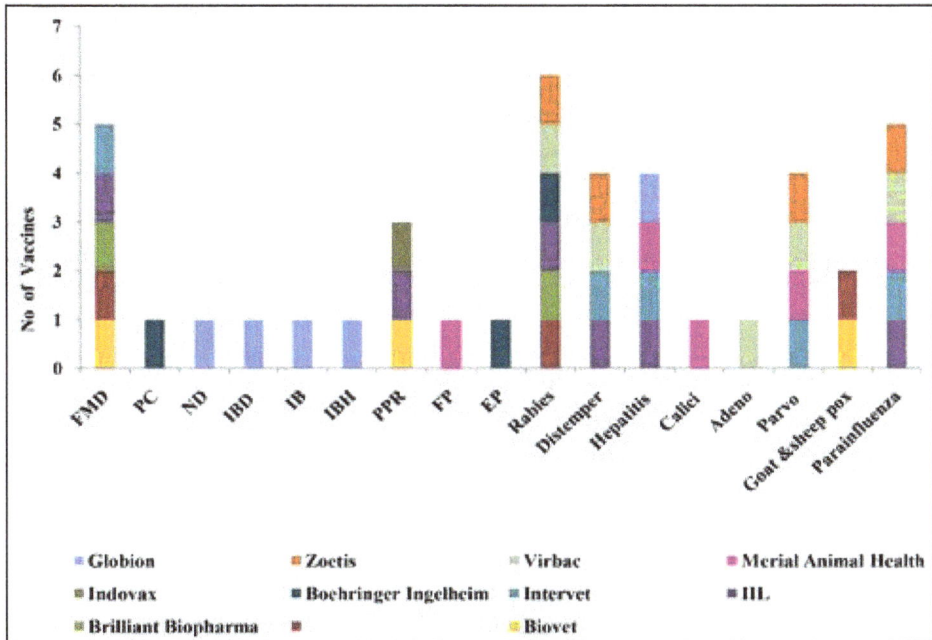

Figure 6.4: Types of Viral Vaccines Available in India.

☆ CPV, CAV and Parainfluenza (5)

☆ Foot and Mouth disease (4)

☆ Of the state owned biologicals, Uttar Pradesh produce 9 vaccines, followed by Maharashtra and Tamil Nadu (7) vaccines

☆ Intervet, IIL, Indovax, Bio-Med and Ventri make most number of the vaccines in that order

6.6 Recombinant Vaccines in India

Though the Indian vaccine manufacturers could establish the vaccine production technologies for conventional vaccines, recombinant vaccines are not licensed so far by any of the Indian companies. Following are some of the recombinant vaccines which are in various stages of development/licensing process.

1. Canary pox vectored canine distemper vaccine: The technology was originally developed by M/s. Merial animal health, USA. Merial was bought by M/s. Sanofi Aventis and Sanofi is trying to licence the vaccine through M/s Sanofi-synthelabo (India) limited in India. The company is trying to licence various combination of canine multi-component vaccines incorporating Canary pox vectored canine distemper. The vaccine is being licensed in the name of **Recombitek** range of vaccines.

2. Turkey Herpesvirus (HVT) vectored IBD vaccine: M/s Sanofi-synthelabo (India) limited is also trying to licence**Vaxxitek HVT +IBD** vaccine which

is a live vaccine against Infectious Bursal Disease and Marek's Disease. The vaccine contains HVT vector with VP2 gene of IBD.

3. Turkey Herpesvirus (HVT) vectored ND vaccine: M/s MSD Animal Health India (Intervet India Ltd) is trying to licence live recombinant Herpesvirus Turkey(HVT) strain containing F gene of Newcastle Virus (NDV) in the name of **Indovax-ND-SB.**

The above three vaccines were available in the market, elsewhere in the world. These vaccines are not available in Indian market so far. However, there are many proven conventional live vaccines are available for the above mentioned diseases. Therefore, these vaccines will not provide any distinct additional advantage over the available conventional vaccines for endemic countries like India.

4. Recombinant oral rabies vaccine: M/s MSD animal health India (Intervet India Ltd) is developing oral rabies vaccine (ORV), **ORA-DPC,** which is derived from SAD B19 rabies virus strain with mutations in glycoprotein and phospho protein genes. This vaccine is under early stages of licensing in India.

5. Recombinant anti-tick vaccine for cattle: Indian Immunologicals Limited had conducted clinical trials for its recombinant mid gut antigen (Bm95) in cattle.

Though the current Indian veterinary vaccine market is not having any recombinant vaccines, there are many research laboratories and institutions are developing such vaccines. India might eventually require such vaccines when they approach the disease eradication stages. In such scenario, recombinant vaccines will provide the ability to differentiate infected animals from vaccinated animals (DIVA) and handling of live agents to prepare the vaccine is also eliminated.

The high cost, stringent regulatory requirement for recombinant vaccines, expertise requirement and need for changing production platform are some of the deterrents for the Indian vaccine industry from embracing the recombinant vaccine production technology.

6.7 Vaccine Manufacturing Plants in India

There are many private and government manufacturers of veterinary vaccines in India. Nine private and 19 government manufacturers are working in India. List of manufacturers are given below. The information about these manufacturers and their vaccines are given in Table 6.2 and Figure 6.5.

Among all manufacturers of veterinary vaccines in India, the Intervet Private Limited is manufacturing highest number of vaccines (19) in Private manufactures and in government manufacturers IVRI is manufacturing highest number of vaccines (9).

6.8 Veterinary Biologicals in India

A few Indian states that do not have their own veterinary vaccine manufacturing

Table 6.2: Private Vaccine Manufacturers

Sl.No.	Manufacturer	Vaccines
1.	Bio-med Pvt. Ltd., Ghaziabad, Uttar Pradesh	IBD, ND, Fowl Pox, Marek's Disease, HS, BQ, ET, Pox, Rabies, ND+IB
2.	Biovet Pvt. Ltd., Kundalahalli, Bangalore	HS, BQ, FMD, PPR
3.	Brilliant bio pharma:, Medak (Dist), Telangana	HS, BQ, ET, Rabies, FMD, HS+BQ
4.	Globion India Private Limited, Secunderabad, Telangana	ND, IBD, Fowl Pox, ND+IB, Fowl Cholera, IB, ND+IB+IBD, Coryza, Hydropericardium
5.	Hester Biosciences Ltd., Ahmedabad, Gujarat, India	ND, IBD, Fowl Pox, Marek's Disease, Pox, ND+IB, PPR, CSF, Brucella
6.	Indian Immunologicals Ltd., Hyderabad, Telangana	HS, BQ, ET, Pox, Rabies, FMD, PPR, HS+BQ, Brucella, FMD+HS, Theileriosis, 6 in 1, CPV, CCV
7.	Indovax Pvt. Ltd., Gurgaon, Haryana	ND, IBD, Fowl Pox, Marek's Disease, ND+IB, Fowl Cholera, IB, IB+ND+IBD, Choryza, Egg Drop Syndrome, Hydropericardium, ND+IBD, ND+IB+IBD+REO, ND+IB+IBD+EDS
8.	Intervet Laboratories Ltd., Pune, Maharashtra	ND, IBD, ET, Rabies, ND+IB, FMD, PPR, HS+BQ, IB, ND+IB+IBD, Coryza, Brucella, 6in 1, ND+IBD, ND+IB+IBD+REO, Mycoplasma Gallisepticum, Bordetella Bronchiseptica + Canine Parainfluenza, Leptospira, Salmonella
9.	Ventri Biologicals, Pune, Maharashtra	ND, IBD, Marek's Disease, ND+IB, Fowl Cholera, ND+IB+IBD, Coryza, ND+IBD, ND+Hydropericardium, Lasota+IBD, Infectious Avian Encephalomyelitis

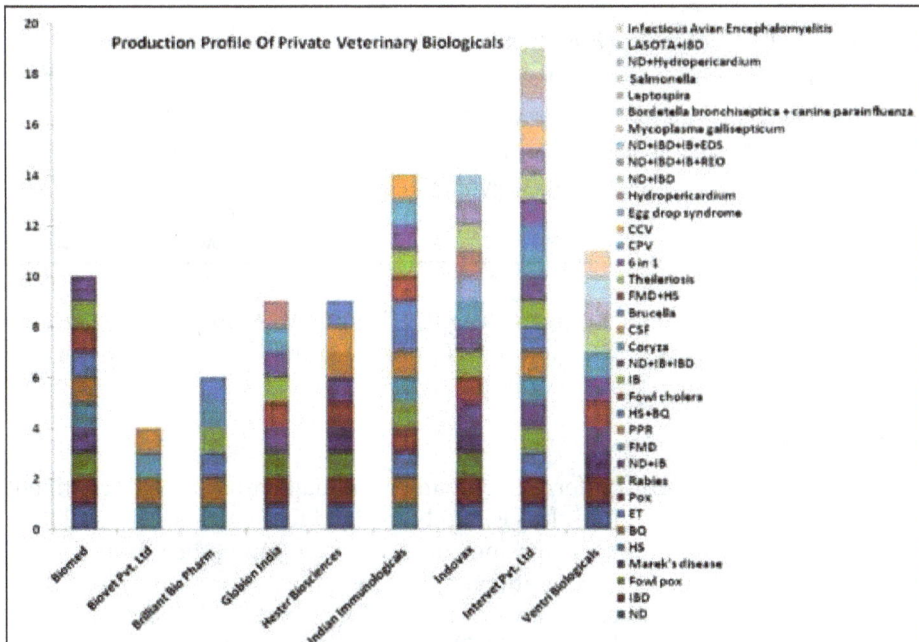

Figure 6.5: Production Profile of Private Veterinary Biologicals.

Table 6.3: Government Vaccine Manufacturers

Sl.No.	Manufacturer	Vaccines
1.	**Animal Vaccine Institute**, Gandhinagar, Gujarat	BQ, HS, ET, ND, SP
2.	**Antirabies Vaccine Laboratory**, Jammu, Jammu and Kashmir	Rabies
3.	**Government of Tamil Nadu,** Institute Ranipet, North Arcot, Tamil Nadu	BQ, HS, Anthrax, ET, ND, SP, Duck Plague
4.	**Haryana Veterinary Vaccine Institute,** Hissar, Haryana	BQ, HS, PPR
5.	**Institute of Animal Health and Biological Production,** Zakura, Jammu and Kashmir	BQ, HS, Anthrax
6.	**Institute of Animal Health and Veterinary Biologicals,** Bangalore, Karnataka	BQ, HS, Anthrax
7.	**Institute of Animal Health and Veterinary Biologicals,** Thiruvananthpuram, Kerala	BQ, HS, Anthrax
8.	**Institute of Animal Health and Veterinary Biologicals,** Mhow, Madhya Pradesh	(BQ, HS, Anthrax, Rabies, CSFV (Lapinised)
9.	**Institute of Animal Health and Veterinary Biologicals,** Calcutta, West Bengal	BQ, HS, Anthrax, Goat Pox
10.	**Institute of Veterinary Biological Products,** Pune, Maharashtra	BQ, HS, Anthrax, ET, SP, Rabies, Brucella
11.	**Institute of Veterinary Biologicals,** Lucknow, Uttar Pradesh	BQ, HS, Anthrax
12.	**Orissa Biological Products Inst. Ltd.,** Buhwaneshwar, Orissa	BQ,HS,Anthrax,ET,Rabies
13.	**Poultry Viral Vaccine Production Centre (P V V P C),** Samalkot, East Godavari, Andhra Pradesh	BQ, HS, Anthrax
14.	**Punjab Veterinary Vaccine Institute,** Punjab Agricultural University Campus, Ludhiana, Punjab	BQ, HS, Rabies
15.	**Regional Veterinary Biologicals Unit**, Jaipur, Rajasthan	BQ, HS, Anthrax
16.	**Institute of Animal Health and Production**, Patna, Bihar	HS, Anthrax
17.	**Institute of Veterinary Biologicals**: Guwahati, Assam	BQ, HS, Anthrax
18	**Veterinary Biologicals and Research Institute,** Hyderabad	BQ, HS, Anthrax
19.	**Indian Veterinary Research Institute (IVRI)**: Bareilly	HS, ET, ND, SP, Brucella, CSFV (Lapinised), PPR, Fowl Pox, Salmonella

institution are Arunachal Pradesh, Nagaland, Sikkim, Manipur, Meghalaya, Jharkhand, Chhattisgarh, Mizoram and Tripura. Figure 6.7 depicts the vaccine manufacturers in different states of India.

6.9 Canine Vaccines

Canines are the most preferred companion animals in Indian sub-continent and the growing urban middle class is highly inclined to own pets. This situation warrants a more serious and increasing concern on the canine health in general and immunization against major pathogens affecting them more specifically. This is well substantiated by recent statistics released in the 19th All India Livestock Census conducted in 2012 (DAHDF, 2012). India has a population of 11.67 million

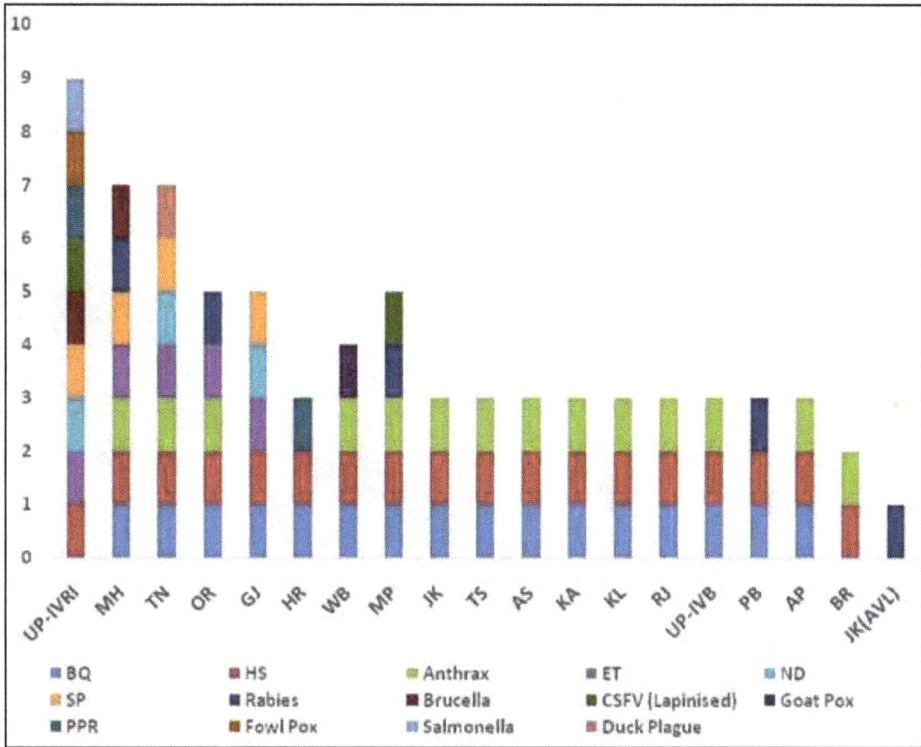

Figure 6.6: Production Profile of State Veterinary Biologicals.

owned dogs excluding 17.13 million community-owned dogs fairly distributed in all the Indian states.

With increased awareness on pet health, several pet health care centres and institutional clinics were established in the recent past. Therefore, the demand for vaccines is on the raise for pets. Additionally, stray dogs act as reservoirs of several viral pathogens and source of acarine/protozoan parasites and the government programs are aiming at reducing the stray dog population and controlling zoonotic diseases like rabies.

The unrestricted movement of the stray dogs with delay in implementation of animal birth control strategies with increasing urbanization in cities exacerbate the present public health setup and may lead to transmission of zoonoses, vector-borne diseases, occupational health hazards and environmental pollution. At present, public health hazards due to urban animal husbandry practices are considerably under-estimated. A recent study conducted in Central India indicated a high level of exposure to various canine viral pathogens such as 88 per cent for Canine Parvo virus, 72 per cent for Canine distemper virus and 71 per cent for Canine adeno virus in free ranging dogs (Belsare *et al.*, 2014).

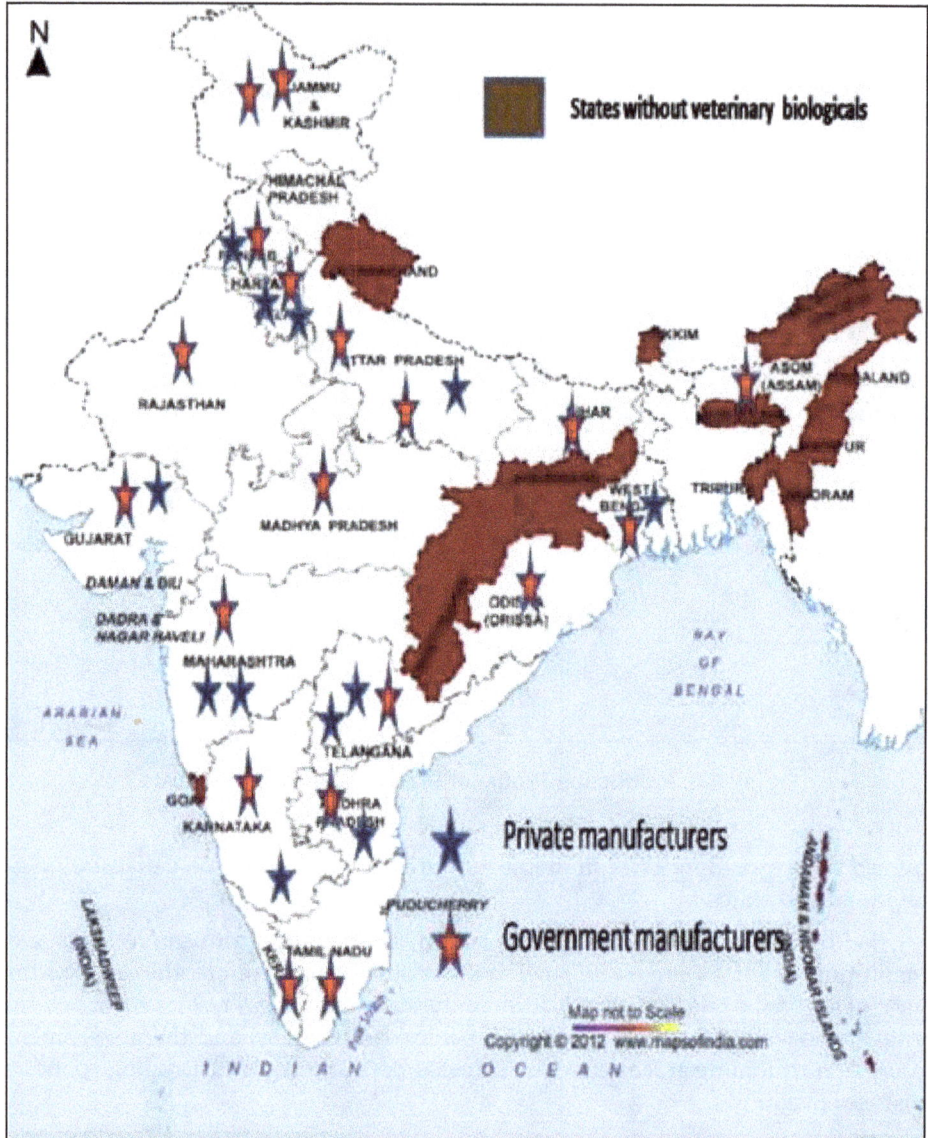

Figure 6.7: State-wise Presence of Veterinary Biologicals in India.

At present of the 24 million canine vaccines are sold annually in India, majority of them are imported vaccines with the exception of a one Indian veterinary vaccine manufacturer and two more manufacturers producing Rabies vaccine alone. All these vaccines contain old and exotic strains. Relevance of these vaccines in controlling the circulating strains of the pathogen is not studied.

Another priority need for India is development of effective anti-fertility vaccine for female dogs that would facilitate the management of stray dogs in urban and rural areas thereby also reducing the burden of rabies infection in the country. This can replace the present surgical intervention which is time consuming and involves a careful post surgical management. Earlier few potential anti-fertility vaccine candidates with Luteinizing hormone releasing hormone in conjugation with Tetanus Toxoid (Ladd *et al.,* 1994) had resulted in immunological castration in 4 weeks of immunization. Recently, Gupta *et al.* (2011) successfully developed protocol for purification of *E. coli* expressed recombinant zona pellucida glycoprotein-3 and found 95 per cent of the mice failed to conceive that received a recombinant fusion protein comprising zona pellucida glycoprotein-3 fragment and gonadotropin releasing hormone.

6.10 Gaps in the existing situation

☆ Only one Indian vaccine manufacturer (Indian Immunologicals Ltd., Hyderabad) produces the complete range of canine vaccines; two other private manufacturers produce rabies vaccines for animals. Most of the canine vaccine demand is met by the imported vaccines.

☆ All the available vaccines use exotic strains and some of the vaccines may not be relevant for Indian context.

☆ There is no systematic study in India for certain diseases like canine corona viral enteritis. However, commercially available combination vaccines contain corona virus component also.

☆ No funding through major funding agencies like ICAR, DAHF, *etc.* except for Animal Birth Control programmes that too at a low priority.

☆ No extensive work on *Brucella canis* and other parasites especially with zoonotic potential.

Some case studies are presented here to show the status of veterinary vaccines market in India. Figure 6.8 and Figure 6.9 shows monthly sales of canine vaccines at Tamil Nadu.

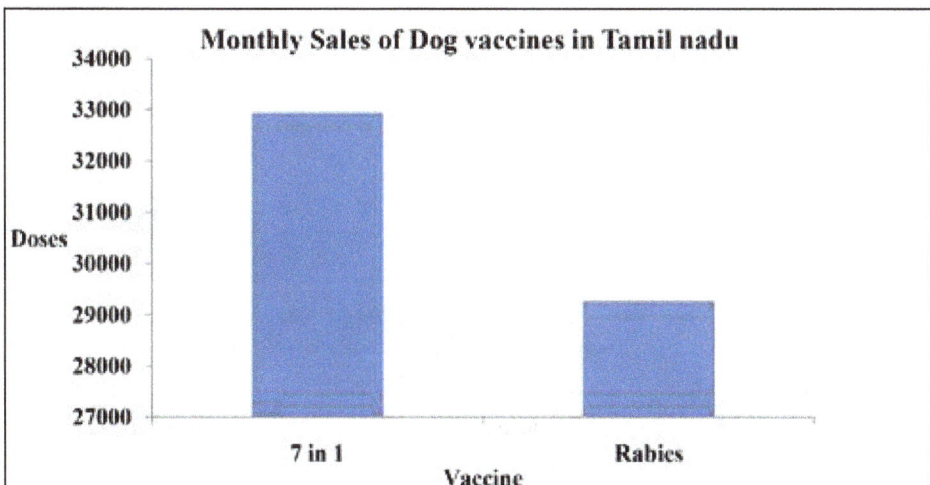

Figure 6.8: Sales of Canine Vaccines in Tamil Nadu.

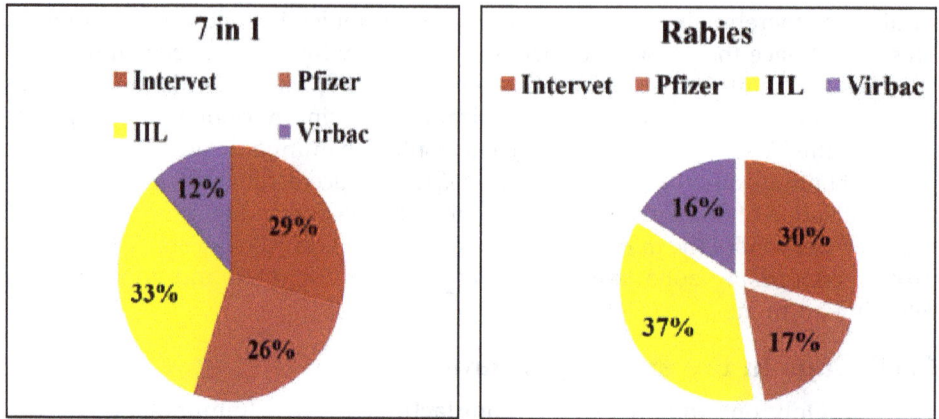

Figure 6.9: Share of different Companies in Sales of Canine Vaccines in Tamil Nadu.

Figure 6.10 and 6.11 showing the sales of different poultry vaccines in Nammakal district of Tamil Nadu.

The maximum sale irrespective of company is NDV followed by Coryza and IB. Ventri biological has the maximum share in the sale of poultry vaccines.

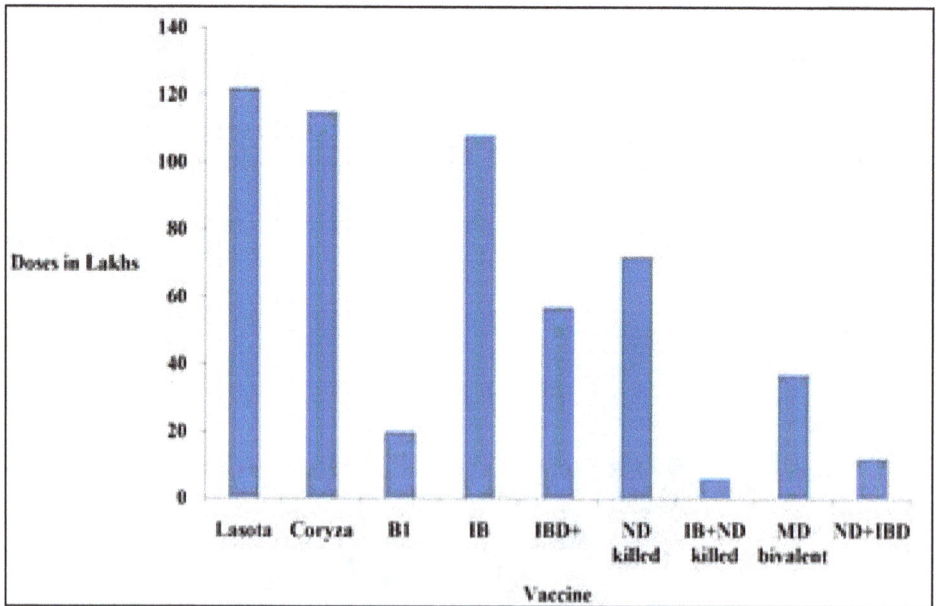

Figure 6.10: Sales of Different Poultry Vaccines at Namakkal.

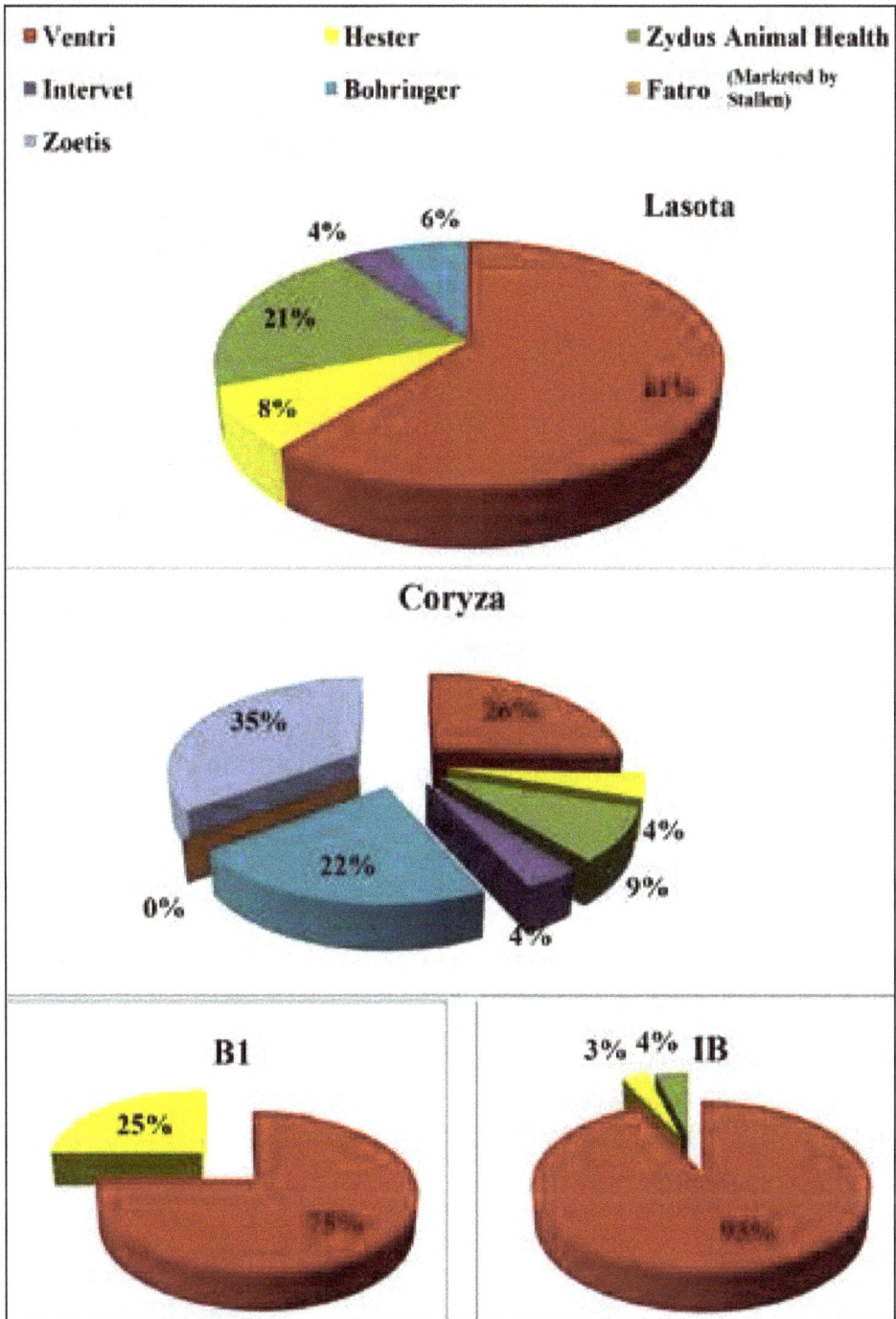

Figure 6.11: Monthly Sales of Poultry Vaccines at Namakkal.
Source: Personal communication from regional sales.

Cost of Vaccines

Table 6.4: Cost of Animal Vaccine from 2010-2016

Species Name	Vaccine	Package Dose	2010 Cost per Dose	2013 Cost per Dose	2016 Cost per Dose
Poultry	RDV-Lasota	200 doses	0.21	0.22	0.21
	RDV-F	200 doses	0.17	0.21	0.21
	IBD Georgia	200 doses	0.88	0.445	0.445
	Fowl Pox	1000 Doses	0.22	0.162	0.173
Sheep and Goats	PPRV	100 Doses	4.08	0.828	3.01
	Sheep pox Vaccine	100 Doses	2.72	0.301	3.04
	ET Vaccine (Inactivated)	50 Doses	1.96	2.5	1.86
	Cl.perfringens vaccine	50 Doses	2.08	2.08	2.08
Bovine	Foot and mouth disease virus vaccine (Inactivated)	15 Doses	10	4.6	10
	Haemorrhagicsepticaemia and black quarter vaccine (Inactivated)	30 Doses	5.45	2.3	6.9
	Anthrax spore vaccine (Live)	50 Doses	10	10.08	10.08
	Foot and mouth disease virus and Haemorrhagicsepticaemia vaccine	30 Doses	4.76	20.4	4.76
Canines	CDV, Canine parvo and para influenza combined vaccine	1 Dose	450	450	450
	CDV, canine parvo vaccine	1 Dose	250	225	250
	Canine Distemper Virus vaccine (Inactivated)	1 Dose	150	375	150
	Canine corona virus vaccine (Killed virus)	1 Dose	250	250	250
	CDV, Parvo and para influenza Live vaccine	1 Dose	300	300	300
	Combined CDV, parvo, adeno virus and para influenza vaccine (Attenuated)	1 Dose	330	330	330
	CD Adenovirus Type-2, Para-influenza Parvovirus Vaccine*	1 Dose	–	–	550
	Combined Canine Distemper Parpovirus Vaccine Live, Freeze Dried*	1 Dose	–	–	400
	Combined CD, Canine Adenovirus Type-2 and Cannine Parvovirus Vaccine*	1 Dose	–	–	450
	Canine parvovirus vaccine (Inactivated)*	1 Dose	–	–	250
	Rabies veterinary vaccine	1 Dose	440	440	440

Contd...

Table 6.4–*Contd...*

Species Name	Vaccine	Package Dose	2010 Cost per Dose	2013 Cost per Dose	2016 Cost per Dose
	Defensor-1 Rabies vaccine (Killed virus)	1 Dose	110	110	110
	Rabies veterinary vaccine (Inactivated)	10 Dose	400	400	400
	Rabies vaccine (Inactivated)	10 Dose	416	416	416
Feline	Feline rhinotracheitis, feline panleukopenia, feline calicivirus, feline pneumonitis (*Chlamydo-philapsittaci*), and feline leukaemia vaccine (Killed virus)	1 dose	410	410	410

* Newly Arrived Vaccines in 2016

Species	Average Cost per Dose		
	FY 2010	*FY 2013*	*FY 2016*
Poultry	0.37	0.25925	0.2595
Sheep	2.71	1.42725	2.4975
Bovine	7.5525	9.345	7.935
Canine	309.6	329.6	309.6

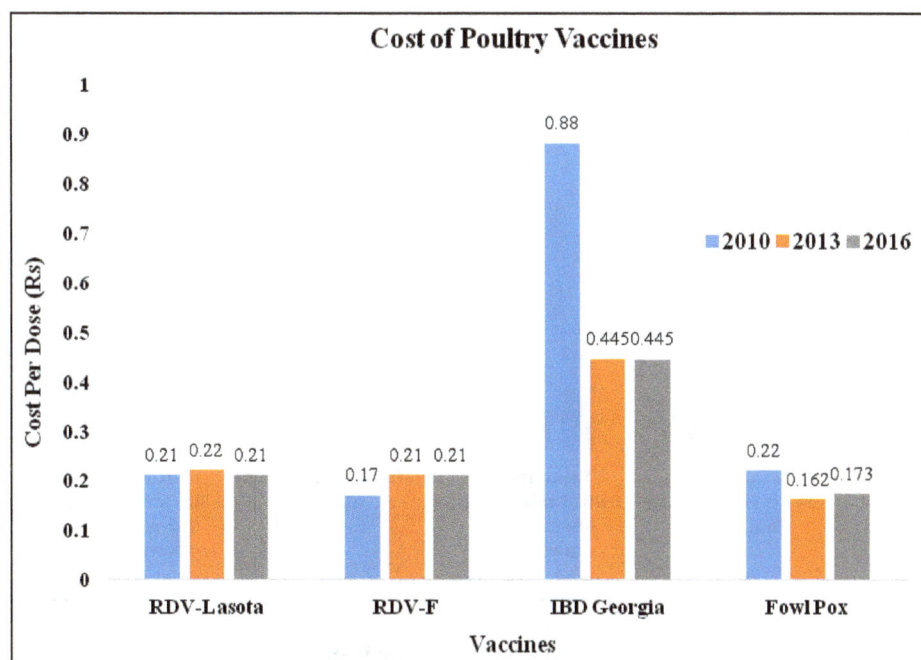

Figure 6.12: Cost of Poultry Vaccine.

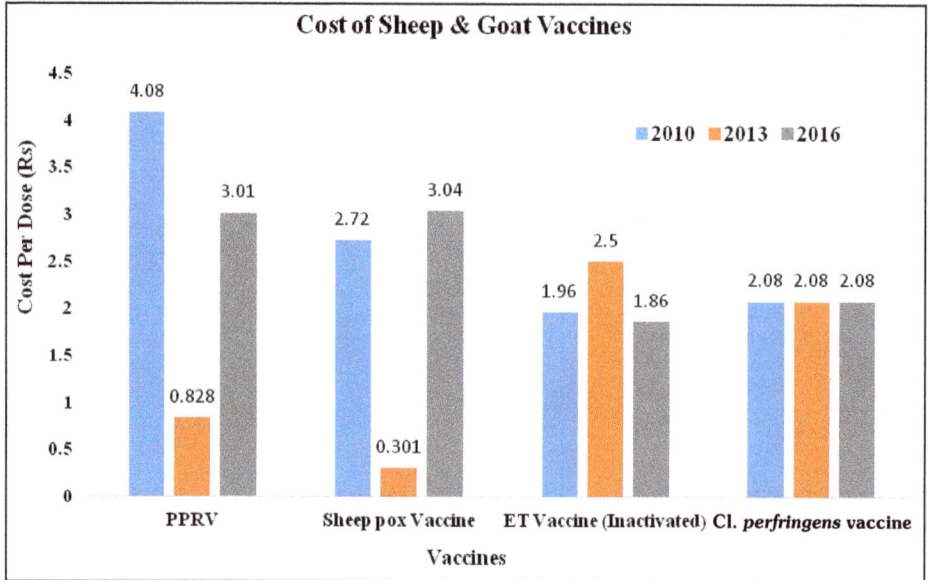

Figure 6.13: Cost of Sheep and Goat Vaccines.

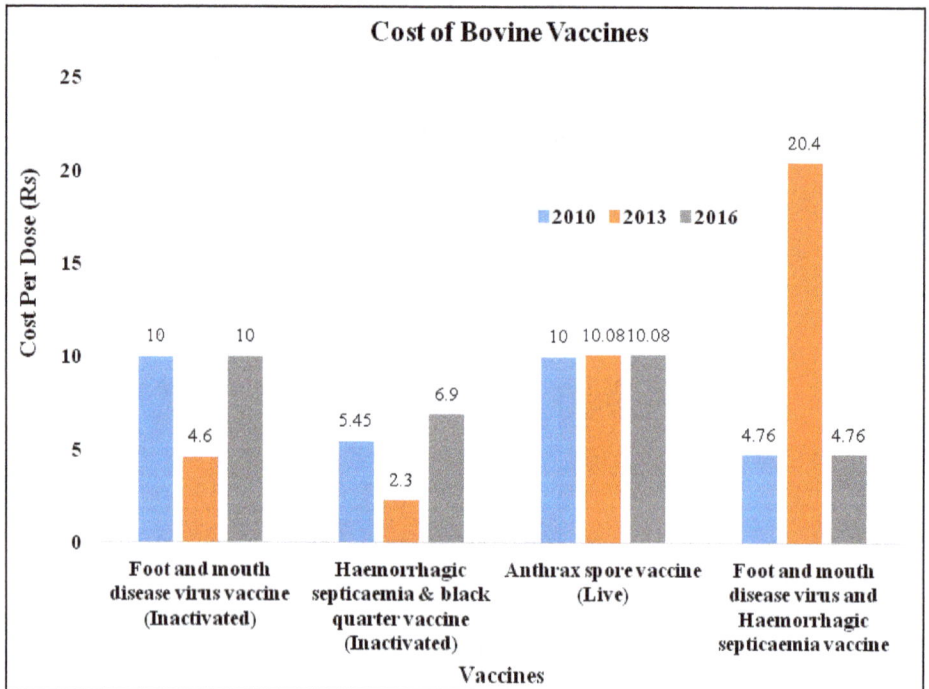

Figure 6.14: Cost of Bovine Vaccines.

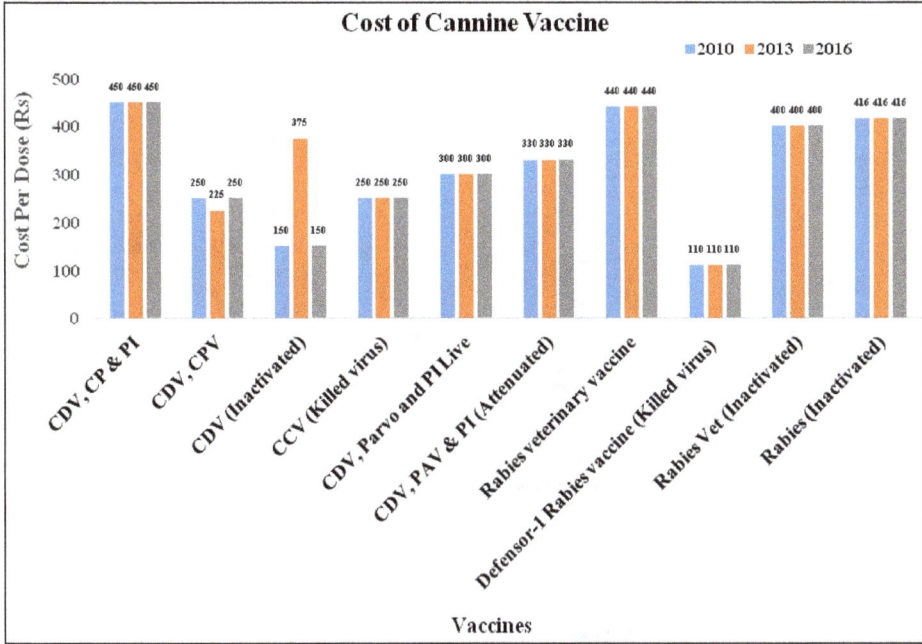

Figure 6.15: Cost of Canine Vaccines.

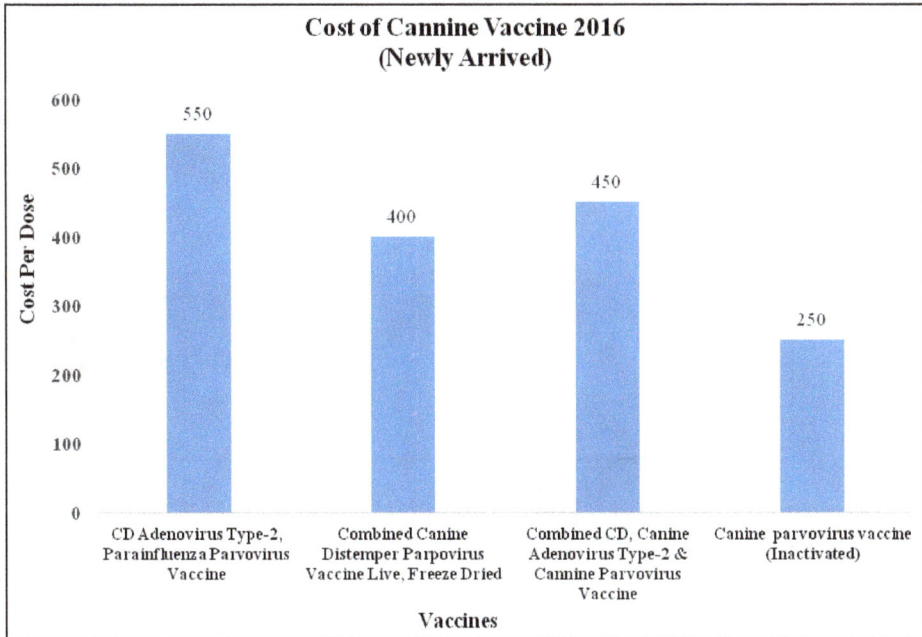

Figure 6.16: Cost of Newly Arrived Canine Vaccines.

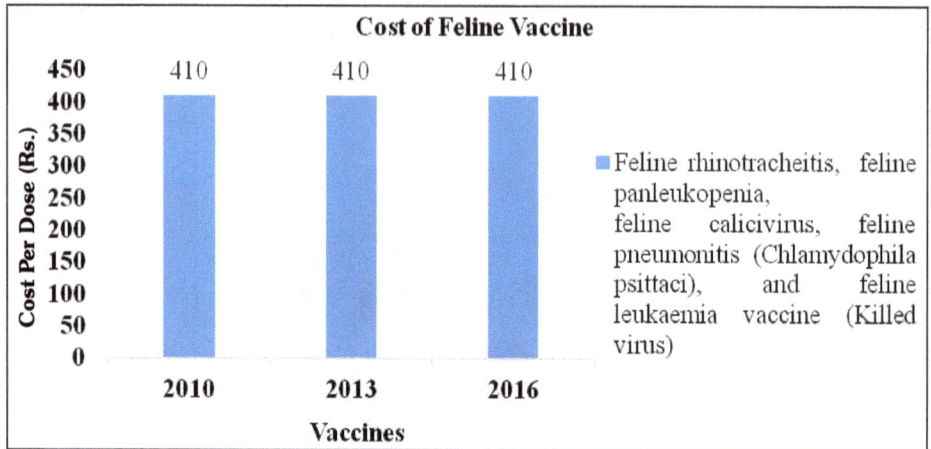

Figure 6.17: Cost of Feline Vaccines.

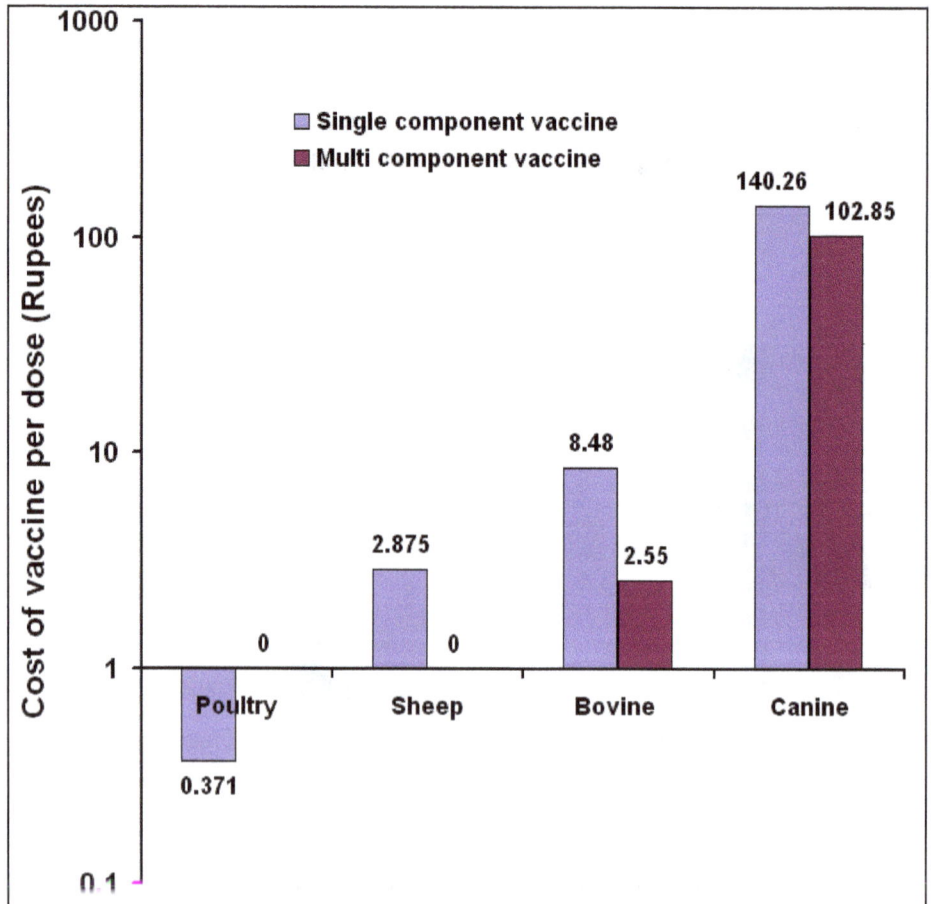

Figure 6.18: Comparison of Single and Multi Dose Vaccines in Market.

☆ The retail cost of veterinary vaccines was analyzed over a period of 6 years (2010 – 2016) and it is very strange that the cost has not changed much.

☆ In fact the average cost per dose of poultry and small ruminant vaccines have reduced marginally, while bovine vaccines have slightly increased and canine vaccines have remained static.

☆ In poultry, IBD vaccine cost has reduced dramatically from 2010 to 2013 to half its price probably due to decreased incidence of this disease during this time frame.

☆ The PPR vaccine cost also reduced dramatically from 2010 to 2013 but has stabilized in 2016. This may be due to more players entering the PPR vaccine market compared to 2010.

☆ Canine vaccines have been introduced in the market lately in 2016 with fewer combinations with either canine parvo or canine distemper along with canine adeno or canine parainfluenza.

☆ Multicomponent vaccines are much cheaper per dose compared to single vaccines.

Some of the main challenges in veterinary vaccine sector are

☆ Cost

☆ Compliance

☆ High initial investments

☆ Less returns

☆ Only government funding for farm animals except poultry and canine

☆ Post vaccination sero surveillance methods

☆ Storage facilities

☆ Lack of consistent demand

☆ Purchase procedures for vaccines through Govt. funding

Some of the methods to combat this challenge in COST of vaccines

☆ Multi component vaccines

☆ Free diagnostics support for purchase of vaccines

☆ Global markets

☆ Clinical Veterinarian should also couple as a diagnostician – This would be possible only with availability of pen side kits

☆ Needle free delivery of vaccines

☆ Larger coverage of animals

☆ Government subsidy

☆ Affordable Veterinary Health Care through NGOs – Welcome Trust, Bill Gates Foundations

References

Belsare A. V., A. T. Vanak and M. E. Gompper. 2014. Epidemiology of Viral Pathogens of Free-Ranging Dogs and Indian Foxes in a Human-Dominated Landscape in Central India. 61 (Suppl. 1): 78–86

Gupta S. K., N. Gupta, P. Suman, S. Choudhury, K. Prakash, T. Gupta, R. Sriraman, S.B. Nagendrakumar, V.A. Srinivasan. 2011. Zona pellucida-based contraceptive vaccines for human and animal utility. Journal of Reproductive Immunology. 88: 240–246

Ladd A, Tsong YY, Walfield AM, Thau R. 1994. Development of an Antifertility Vaccine for Pets Based on Active Immunization against Luteinizing Hormone-Releasing Hormone. Biology of Reproduction. 51:1076–1083.

7

Diagnosis of Animal Diseases: Understanding Challenges and Limitations

7.1 History of Diagnosis

The Oxford dictionary defines "Diagnosis" as the act of discovering or identifying by examination the exact cause of an illness or a problem. It originated from the Greek word literally meaning "to discern or to distinguish or to know thoroughly.

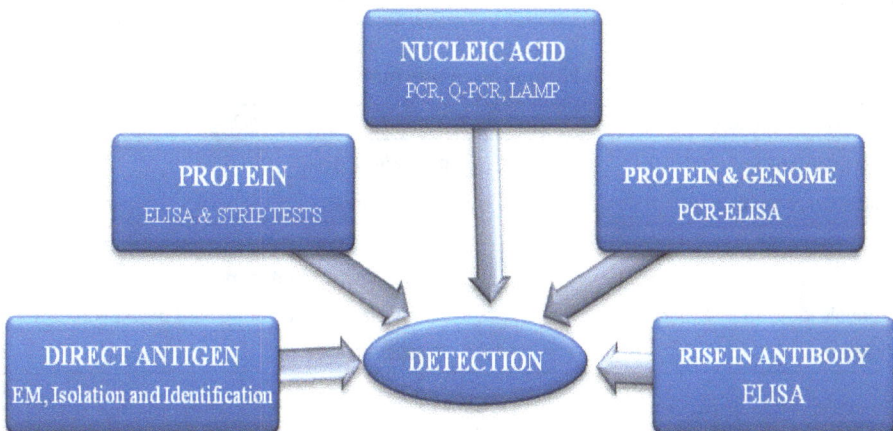

7.2 Protein vs. Genome Based Diagnostics

An immunoassay is an analytical method, quantitative or qualitative which uses antibodies as reagents to quantitate specific analytes. Immunoassays rely absolutely on the specificity and affinity of the interaction between epitope and paratope.

They offer something completely different from the polymerase chain reaction (PCR). Both these techniques rely on interaction between two complementary sequences, linked to signal generation. Both can also involve an amplification step and can be either qualitative or quantitative. Both these technologies provide complementary information.

Table 7.1: Comparison of Immunoassays and PCR

Immunoassays	*PCR*
Provide information on protein	Provide information on DNA/mRNA
Possible to detect conformation and sequence	Detects only sequence
Can also be applicable for haptens such as steroid and thyroid hormones	Only for nucleic acids
May or may not correlate with mRNA levels	Higher mRNA levels do not necessarily mean higher protein levels
Neutralization of biological activity based assays possible	Not possible

Table 7.2: Lab Based vs. Field Based Diagnostics

Lab-Based Diagnostics	*Field Based Diagnostics*
More sensitive	Less sensitive
More cumbersome to perform/time consuming	Easy to perform
More reliable	Less reliable
Confirmatory test	Screening test
Assay based	Kit based
Needs equipments and expertise	All self contained

Table 7.3: Human vs. Veterinary Diagnostics

Human Diagnostics	*Veterinary Diagnostics*
Better affordability	Poor affordability
Application of technology	Naïve market
Mass production	Limited requirement
Individual based	Herd based (except for pets)
Diagnosis leads to treatment	Diagnosis leads to control and prevention
Single entity	Multiple etiology

7.3 Diagnostic Test vs. Screening Tests

A diagnostic test is used to determine the presence or absence of a disease when a subject shows signs or symptoms of the disease

A screening test identifies asymptomatic individuals who may have the disease

The diagnostic test is performed after a positive screening test to establish a definitive diagnosis

7.4 Ruling in or Ruling Out a Disease

The selection of an appropriate diagnostic test depends upon the intended use of the results. If the intention is to rule out a disease, reliable negative results are required for which a test with high sensitivity (*i.e.* few false negatives) is used. If it is desired to confirm a diagnosis or find evidence of disease (*i.e.* to "rule in" the disease) we require a test with reliable positive results (*i.e.* high specificity). As a general rule of thumb, a test with at least 95 per cent sensitivity and 75 per cent specificity should be used to rule out a disease and one with at least 95 per cent specificity and 75 per cent sensitivity used to rule in a disease (Pfeiffer, 1998).

7.5 Diagnosis of Disease vs. Infection

Infection is the invasion, multiplication and host response of an organism by disease causing agents.

A disease is an abnormal clinical manifestation or illness resulting from an infection.

Infections usually result in disease, but not always. Disease is the end result of an infection.

An animal is having infection with tuberculosis (TB) if it is infected with pathogenic of organisms *Mycobacterium* species.

But the animal would suffer from the disease TB only when the immune system is not able to control the organism and then the animal would become sick.

While a skin test would indicate that the animal is infected, an abnormal chest X ray or isolation of organism would indicate active infection.

Ideally a diagnostic test should classify all subjects who have the disease as "diseased" and vice versa. This ability of the test under question to classify subjects is evaluated before the test is applied in diagnosis

The field of diagnostics has evolved over the years for instance bacteria were identified through phenotypic and cultural characters. This was followed by protein based method such as ELISA used for serological characterization. With the advent of PCR, nucleic acid based detection methods have overwhelmed the earlier technologies due to its speed, sensitivity and discriminating power. While the conventional microbiologist would still adhere to the isolation and identification of the etiological agent as a confirmatory diagnostic method this may no longer be sustainable in all cases and in all context where the genome based diagnostic method are far superior in terms of sensitivity. Application of this technology in a clinical diagnostic setting is fraught with limitation due to its increased sensitivity. A small aerosol contamination of the amplified product from earlier samples would lead to false positive misdiagnosis with tremendous adverse effect to the patient.

Every diagnostic platform tries to solve an earlier problem at least in one respect but ends up creating a newer problem. The quest of science is to keep identifying this problem and finding out ways to overcome them. Typical example is in the case of PCR and its modifications such as multiplex PCR, nested PCR *etc.*, each with its distinct advantages. However PCR was a qualitative method through which quantification of genome was not possible. Then the invention of real time PCR with its various chemistries converted PCR into a quantitative method. Although real time PCR is a 'state-of-art' method used in various diagnostic laboratory especially with the probe method which overcomes the laboratory contamination and non specific amplification is still remain costly and require huge infra structure facility although it is widely used in human medicine for the diagnosis of swine flu, chikungunya, dengue, *etc.* The cost of testing per sample varies from Rs. 2,000/- to Rs. 8,000/-. The use of this technology in veterinary medicine in countries like India would be rather limited only to the apex laboratory of this state.

Another extrapolation of the PCR was the loop mediated isothermal amplification which overcame the need for repeated thermal cycling and gel electrophoresis of the amplified product. Since its introduction in 2001 LAMP has been applied for the detection of almost all the known bacterial, viral and parasitic pathogens. However the high amplification efficiency along with the high stability of the amplified products produces false positive reaction in the laboratory following its routine application for a limited period of time.

One another disadvantage of PCR was whether the amplified product came from a live infectious organism or a dead non-infectious organism. This problem has been overcome by the introduction of viability PCR wherein a dye is used to label the organisms which are then exposed to laser light. The dye enters only the dead organism and binds to its DNA and upon exposure to laser light the DNA is cleaved making it un-amplifiable there by whatever amplification seen in PCR is from the live organism, This search for newer technologies overcoming the disadvantage of earlier technologies and solving or reducing the issue of the created technology would go on.

In the context of protein based diagnostic platforms, ELISA and Lateral flow assays (LFA) have stormed diagnostic market especially in the veterinary sector. Various type of ELISA such as Indirect ELISA, Competitive ELISA, Immuno Capture ELISA is commonly used as kits. Upon careful examination, it has been found that most of the ELISA used for vaccine efficacy studies is based on Indirect ELISA mostly using the whole antigen. For example poultry kits for Newcastle Disease Virus, Infectious bursal disease virus, Infectious bronchitis virus use purified whole virus antigen for coating the ELISA plate.

There are very few kits using recombinant defined antigen although several published studies are available using various gene targets. Whether this is due to the ease of cultivation and purification of the viruses mostly in embryonated eggs as opposed to expression and purification of recombinant protein or due to the better performance of the kit with whole virus antigen are not known although we may believe that the former is the reason. Most of the ELISA kits quantify the serum response in terms of titres and has an interface with software support to convert the ELISA OD's into titres along with interpretations. Although in many cases protection titres are not given the increase or decrease in titres following vaccination helps the user to generate a flock profile with respect to the antibody status in the breeding flocks. Most of this kit also come with precoated plates and stabilized substrate which enables ELISA to be performed in 2 to 3 steps. However the cost of this kit in Indian context per sample is still high and there is a scope for huge reduction in cost if these kits are made indigenously.

Most of the disease diagnostic kits are mostly Competitive ELISA based. The specificity of the kits is being achieved by the monoclonal antibody used. The competitive ELISA based kits has better correlation with the serum neutralization titres if the monoclonal antibody used is against a immune dominant neutralizing epitope of the antigen. OIE approved kits for peste des petits ruminants (PPR) and Bluetongue are competitive ELISA based.

Immuno capture ELISA is mostly used for the detection of the antigen by the use of monoclonal antibody against different epitopes on the antigen. The choice of this pair is very critical that determines the sensitivity of the assay.

The LFA are a handy test to be used in the field without the need of any technical expertise and results being read in 5 to 10 minutes. This assay also works on the principle of Immuno capture ELISA but without the need for any substrate reaction. The colored line seen in the LFA is due to localization of colloidal gold/color latex particle in a narrow zone. Although this test is very rapid and field based the sensitivity of the assay is largely compromised by the short time for the antigen-antibody reaction. So although many LFA commercial kits are available caution has to be exercised in applying this kit due to poor sensitivity and the interpretation has to be contextual.

There is always a doubt whether the diagnostic assays have to fulfill the market need or the research output should create a market for itself. In other words 'mind to market' or 'market to mind' is the strategy that needs to be employed. It appears that we should have a bit of both. If the market to mind strategy comes up with a path breaking technology with several advantages over the existing one then a market would be created for it. However if the technology is known proven one which is being applied in a newer area, then the market survey for its requirement may be needed to drive commercialization.

New path-breaking technologies such as different methods of LFA, micro fluidic based diagnostic system or fluorescence polarized assays are the likely future.

Why Assays end up in Deep Freezers and not in Market Shelves?

☆ Technologies always keep changing

☆ Lack of continuity in research/personnel

☆ Changing priority – dictated by funding

☆ Lack of drive and zeal on the part of the inventor

☆ No support for validation – validating agency acceptance (*especially free of cost or if they need it*)

Challenges for the Veterinary Diagnostician

☆ Cost

☆ Is treatment going to change?

☆ Ultimatum – sell or slaughter of the animal – Greater economic burden if diagnostic costs involved

☆ Poor reproducibility of assays

☆ Approved methodology

☆ Need of technical expertise – for performance and interpretation

☆ Few tests only in the form of kits

☆ Mindset of the end user in terms of confirmatory or lab based diagnosis

The Way Forward

☆ **Identification of need** (Time elapse between identification, development of a assay/kit/commercialization – would the need be same after such a prolonged incubation)

☆ **Technology improvement** in terms of expertise – collaboration with people who know it, such as protein chemist

☆ **Diagnosis with relevance to humans also**

☆ **Awareness among practicing vets to confirm clinical diagnosis using laboratory tests**

☆ **Aiming for Global markets** - *Extensive validation*

☆ **Link with industry before development** (*for this industry should have faith in the capability of the institution/inventor*)

Future of Veterinary Laboratory Diagnosis

☆ Market surveys for need of a kit

☆ Use standardized reagents such as scFv or recombinant antigens (*This would ensure reproducibility*)

☆ Molecular diagnosis with appropriate internal controls and stringent quality checks

☆ Novel innovative approaches

☆ Medical Instrumentation support

☆ Translational support in terms of research resources – inbred lines, SPF eggs, linkages, infrastructure and regulatory support, biotechnology means for mass production *etc.*

In short,

☆ Clinical diagnosis – user based: The bottom-line of any treatment is to save the life or the productivity of the animal. If the veterinarian assures this, then the owner is ready to spend the money on diagnosis and treatment. Hence he is willing to pay for the same !

☆ Epidemiological diagnosis – Govt. agency based: An epidemiological diagnosis is not likely to benefit the animal owners directly. For instance whether sheep/goat are affected by sheep pox/PPR/Bluetongue is immaterial to its owner. All (s)he would be interested is to know from the Veterinarian whether the animal can be saved. If not, the owner would have to decide on the sacrifice of the animal and redeem what little (s)he can. In such cases, the owner of the animal would not be keen to pay for the diagnostics which may ultimately benefit the State in the control or epidemiology of the disease for which the Government may have to pay and sponsor the diagnostics cost.

7.6 Veterinary Diagnostics

In the field of diagnostics the international key players are IDEXX Laboratories (U.S.), VCA Antech Inc. (U.S.), Abaxis Corporation (U.S.), Heska Corporation (U.S.), Zoetis Inc. (U.S.), Mindray Medical (China), Neogen Corporation (U.S.), and Thermo Fisher Scientific Inc. (U.S.). Figure 7.1 depicts the leading region of veterinary diagnostics globally, although the growing companion animal population coupled with the positive development towards animal health expenses has led to the outsized market share of the North American and European market. However, the Asia- Pacific region such as India and China is slated to show a significant growth during the forecast period represents the highest growth opportunity for the market during the forecast period of 2013 to 2018.

The global market for animal therapeutics and diagnostics market is predicted to grow substantially over the next few years from just over $2,859 Million in 2013 to approximately $4,200 Million by 2018 with a CAGR of 7.2 per cent. North America and Europe are the major leaders with nearly 45 per cent and 30 per cent share respectively. Increasing companion animal population, coupled with the positive trend towards animal health spending has led to an increased market of these regions. The Asia-Pacific region is expected to have the highest growth opportunity

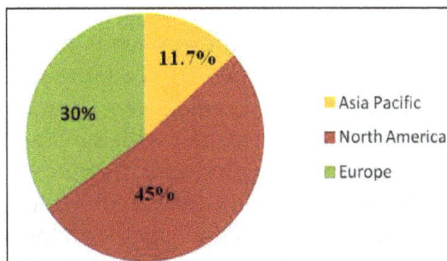

Figure 7.1: Key Regions of Veterinary Diagnostics.
Source: www.marketsandmarkets.com.

for the Veterinary diagnostics market with a CAGR of 11.7 per cent due to increasing livestock and companion animal population in the region, growing awareness about animal health, and rising per capita expenditure on animal health.

Globally the top eight major players in the veterinary diagnostics market mentioned above collectively accounted for nearly 75 per cent of the global veterinary diagnostics market in 2012. Indian veterinary market with the presence of companies like Virbac Animal Health India, Cadila, Concept Pharma, Intas Pharmaceuticals, Pfizer Inc, Novartis AG and Wockhardt Ltd and many others, in manufacturing of veterinary drugs or vaccines, has fewer players in veterinary diagnostic market in India.

Diagnostic industry predominantly comprises of three groups of players that include small specialist labs, larger life sciences companies and instrumentation companies. The small labs are involved in the development of test kits, reagents for veterinary diseases; the larger life sciences companies are competitive on more developed test kit markets and the instrumentation companies leverage their existing technologies with capability to re-purpose clinical human analyzers to customize for the veterinary market. The veterinary analyzers are largely positioned for companion animal clinics while small laboratories and larger life science companies positioned for food animal diagnostics market for infectious and zoonotic diseases.

Abaxis with next generation diagnostic technology has entered the global veterinary diagnostics market dominated by IDEXX Laboratories and VCA Antech. The product portfolio of Abaxis includes POC kits (lyme, parvo, heartworms, ehrlichia, avian influenza, etc.), Hematology analyzer (a comprehensive 22 parameter complete blood picture with cellular histograms) and specialty analyzers with multiple panels to choose from for various tests and assays. Their products are distributed globally but not currently available in India.

Product Development

Diagnostics play a pivotal role in contributing disease control planning, as it creates value chain mapping of diseases with subsequent risk assessment of disease surveillance. Appropriate drug use and other disease control strategies depend on correct diagnosis and working understanding of the suitability of therapeutic options.

The growth of the veterinary diagnostics over the past few years can be attributed to launch of numerous products with adaptation of technologies from the human diagnostics platform into the veterinary diagnostics segment and this trend is expected to continue and grow further with the human diagnostics getting cheaper. The product development in veterinary diagnostics industry is along the lines of either animal infectious disease tests or core test analyzers (*e.g.* clinical chemistry, hematology) and molecular diagnostics with the molecular diagnostics platforms growing the fastest due to high revenues with use of techniques such as real time PCR, micro fluidics and next generation sequencing. The products and technologies from diagnostic product developers lack aggressive awareness creation among clinicians or do not cater to unmet needs in diagnosis sector. This could be due to lack of established commercialization pathway, need of champions to drive the product commercialization, lack of public sector initiation and commercialization models such as risk sharing models for validation studies.

Growth Drivers

The overall growth of this industry is mainly attributed to the growing incidences of animal disease outbreaks, increasing incidences of zoonotic diseases, increasing companion animal market backed by the rise in the adoption of pets, increase of disposable incomes and the advancements in the veterinary diagnostics industry. Highly organized livestock and poultry sectors, increased awareness towards prevention of diseases and as an assistance tool in livestock management practices are expected to fuel the demand for diagnostic tests.

Constraints

Although there are immense opportunities for growth in the veterinary diagnostic sector, most of the kits are not customized to regional requirements, lacking specificity and sensitivity in the test results. The other barrier for growth is the cost of the kits for as the customer is highly price sensitive. Affordable and easy to use disease diagnostics are of immense demand and indicate a potential market opportunity for the manufacturers along with a need for expansion of public procurement programs and distribution mechanism to trigger private sector companies' engagement in production along with adoption in farms. Though the price is of constraint in this sector, the current technologies are associated with challenges in accurate diagnosis due to low specificity and sensitivity with a need for expert intervention to perform and interpret the results. The limited number of experts, veterinary practitioners in the country also hinder the growth of the diagnostic sector. In addition, disease treatments are not accessible to smallholder farmers (*e.g.*, due to high cost, inaccessible regions, *etc.*).

License approval by the regulatory bodies with respect to the procedural matters and timelines also deter entry of players to the veterinary diagnostics. For *e.g.* Zoetis faced licensing hurdles with the Salmonellosis diagnosis kit which has triggered its partnership with Hester for its distribution. The fragmented animal industry would require ingenuity on commercial models and strategic partnerships with smaller companies having product development capabilities. With these constraints, market heads towards adopting more preventive strategies such as vaccinations observed in the poultry sector due to higher costs of treatment vs. diagnostics.

7.7 Livestock Diagnostics

Currently the livestock diagnostics is done in public reference laboratories with high turnaround time. There is a need for capacity expansion to reduce lead time for appropriate specialist/veterinarian intervention for treatment. The national vaccine programs have also led to an increased awareness and a need for point of care diagnostic kits, *e.g.*, NIVEDI kits for Brucellosis diagnosis have high potential with low cost that could cater to large volumes. But the kits are not readily available due to manufacturing constraints of the institute. The same is the case for PPR diagnostics supplied by IVRI, Mukteswar. These kits are not shipped and need to be collected in person. Future trends indicate the need in product development for Mastitis, Brucellosis, pregnancy detection, theileriosis, PPR, CSF diagnostic kits for livestock.

7.8 Poultry Diagnostics

In poultry, the market adopts various strategies for preventing the diseases rather than treatment as mentioned earlier due to higher diagnostics costs in comparison to the vaccinations. Although stamping and culling is the preferred practice for diseased birds over poultry diagnostics. Poultry diagnostic services are taken up by institutes such as Poultry Disease Diagnosis and Surveillance Laboratory (PDDSL), Project Directorate on Poultry (PDP), Avian disease diagnostic labs of State Universities and service of commercial poultry companies such as Suguna and Venkateshwara Hatcheries with no much need in product development.

7.9 Companion Animals

As per the reports, the companion diagnostics market is still nascent, and it is projected to reach $3.5 billion by 2020 from a base value of $1.1 billion in 2013, growing at a CAGR of 20 per cent during 2014 to 2020. Currently, the companion animal diagnostics is commonly carried out in large veterinary clinics and human diagnostic laboratories. A few POCT kits are imported that are highly priced, have low specificity and sensitivity leading to low acceptance and adoption by the veterinary clinicians. With the increasing growth of pet animal population along with a willingness to spend by pet owners on their well-being and willingness to use by the veterinarians, there is immense need and opportunity to develop numerous diagnostic kits for this segment of animals such as diagnosis of Leptospirosis, Parasiticides, Canine distemper, skin diseases *etc.*

7.10 Indian Scenario

Three major players are present in the Indian context for veterinary diagnostics manufacturers in India as depicted in Figure 7.2.

Two major suppliers of imported kits are M/s. Adinath Veterinary Products Pvt. Ltd., one of the leading distributors of animal disease diagnostic kits from eighteen principal companies and M/s. Grace scientific is the leading distributors of diagnostics and biotechnology related products.

7.11 Availability of Diagnostic Kits for Animals

Figure 7.3-7.6 represents the total available kits for diseases diagnosis of bovine, canine, avian and swine and diagnostic platforms.

7.12 Different Platforms for Veterinary Diagnostic Kits

7.12.1 Lateral Flow Assay

Lateral flow assays (LFAs) are point-of-care (POC) devices currently used for qualitative and semi- quantitative diagnosis in non-laboratory settings. The parts of

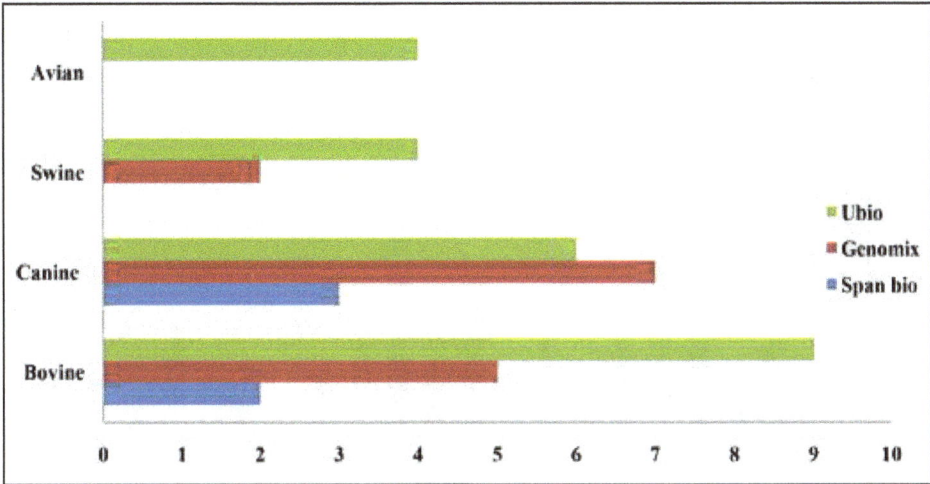

Figure 7.2: Major Players of Indian Veterinary Diagnostics.

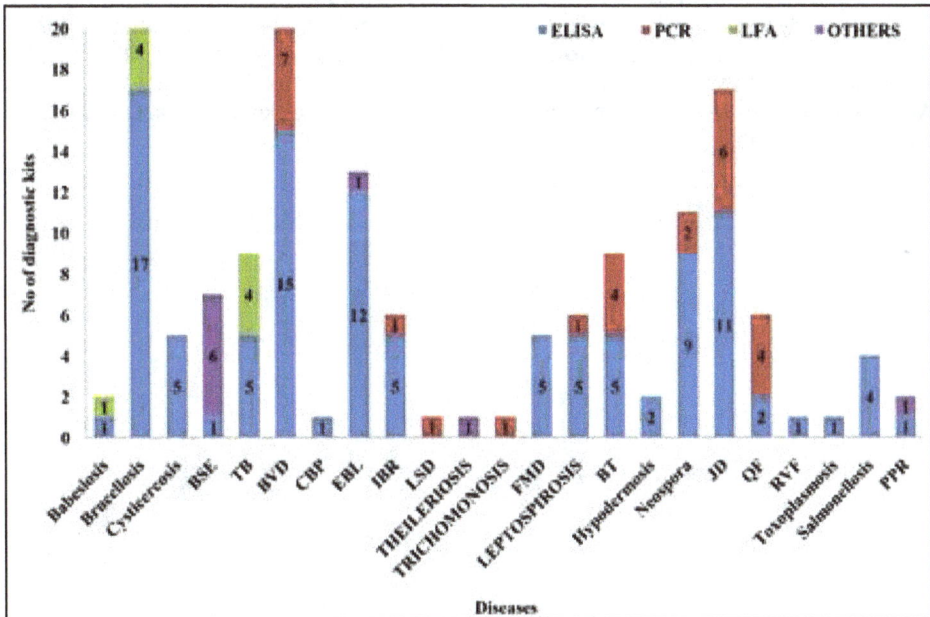

Figure 7.3: Availability of diagnostics kits for ruminant diseases

BSE: Bovine Spongiform Encephalopathy; TB: Tuberculosis; BVD: Bovine Viral Diarrhea; CBPP: Contagious Bovine Pleuropneumonia; EBL: Enzootic Bovine Leukosis; IBR: Infectious Bovine Rhinotracheitis; LSD: Lumpy Skin Diseases; FMD: Foot and Mouth disease; BT: Bluetongue; JD: Johne's Disease; QF: Q fever; RVF: Rift Valley Fever; PPR: Peste des Petits Ruminants.

Others: Agglutination test, AGID: Agar gel immunodiffusion.

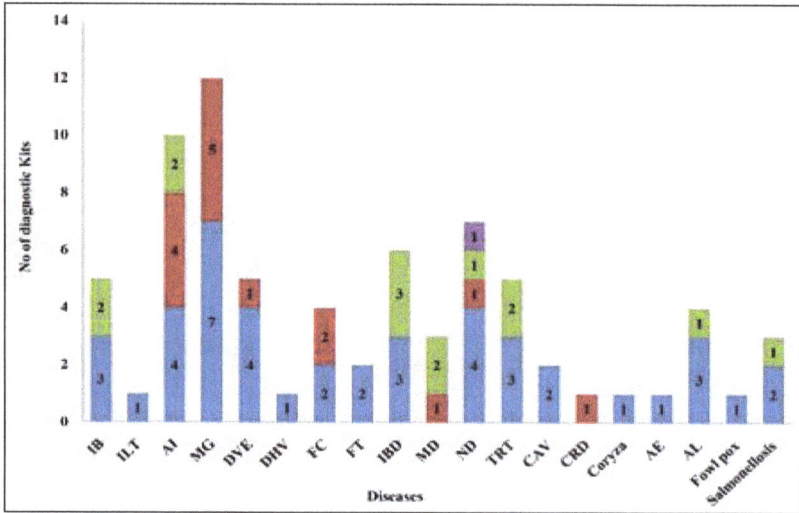

Figure 7.4: Availability of Diagnostic Kits for Avian Diseases.

IB: Infectious Bronchitis; ILT: Infectious Laryngotracheitis; AI: Avian Influenza; MG: Avian Mycoplasmosis; DVE: Duck Virus Enteritis; DHV: Duck Hepatitis Virus; FC: Fowl cholera; FT: Fowl typoid; IBD: Infectious Bursal Diseases; MD: Marek's Diseases; ND: Newcastle Disease; TRT: Turkey Rhinotracheitis; CAV: Chicken Anemia Virus; AE: Avian Encephalomyelitis; ALV: Avian Leukosis Virus. Others: Card agglutination test.

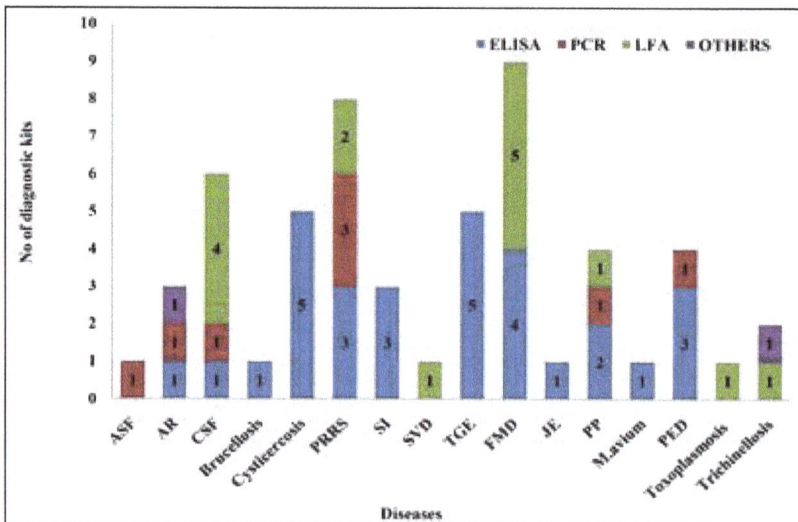

Figure 7.5: Availability of Diagnostics Kits for Swine Diseases.

ASF: African Swine Fever; AR: Atrophic Rhinitis; CSF: Classical Swine Fever; PRRS: Porcine Reproductive and Respiratory Syndrome; SI: Swine Influenza; TGE: Transmissible Gastroenteritis; FMD – Foot and Mouth Disease; JE: Japanese encephalitis; PPV: Porcine Parvo; PED: Porcine Epidemic Diarrhoea. Others: CAT: card agglutination test.

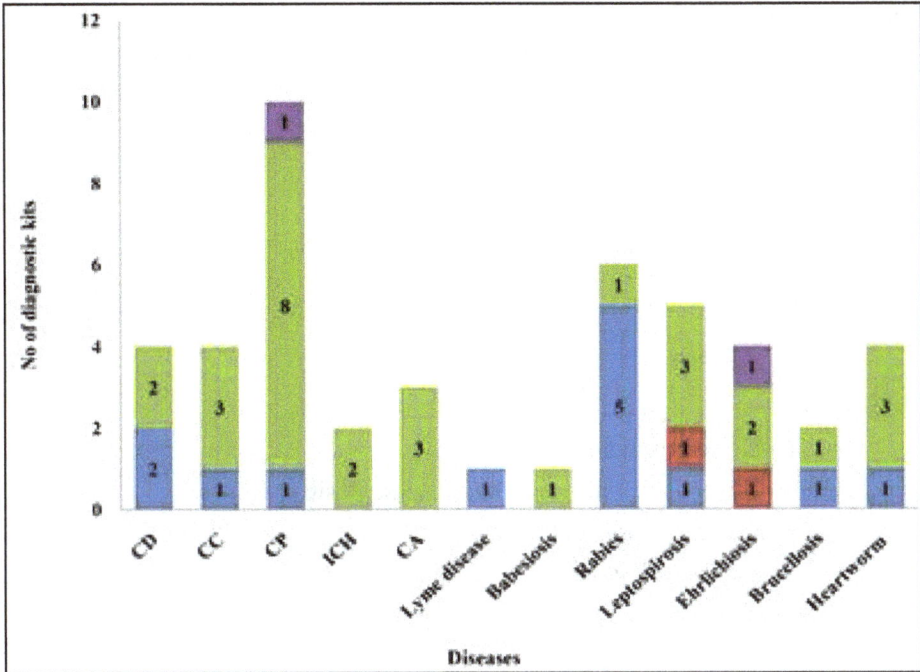

Figure 7.6: Availability of Diagnostic Kits for Canine Diseases.
CD: Canine Distemper; CC: Canine Corona; CP: Canine Parvo; ICH: Infectious Canine Hepatitis; CA: Canine Adeno. Others: CAT: Card agglutination test.

a LFA include sample application pad, conjugate pad, nitrocellulose membrane and adsorption pad. Nitrocellulose membrane is imprinted with test and control lines. Pre-immobilized reagents on the LFA become active upon flow of liquid sample and buffer inducing immune complex formation. Since one of the reagents is coupled with a reporter dye such as coloured latex or colloidal gold, concentration of this tagged reagent in a narrow zone exhibits itself as a colored line.

The advantages of LFA include:

☆ One step analysis

☆ Rapid

☆ User friendly

☆ No instrumentation required

☆ Long term stability

The disadvantages include low sensitivity since the time for the immune reaction to take place is very short and results are qualitative or at best semi-quantitative.

7.12.2 Polymerase Chain Reaction (PCR)

PCR is an enzymatic amplification method that permits amplification of a exact

DNA fragment from a complex pool of DNA. PCR can be performed using DNA from various sources including tissues, microbes, fluid samples, swabs, semen *etc.* Only trace amounts of DNA is required for PCR.

Advantages

- ☆ Quick
- ☆ Reliable
- ☆ Sensitive
- ☆ Relatively easy
- ☆ Specific

Limitations

- ☆ Need for equipment
- ☆ Aerosol Contamination leading to false positive results
- ☆ Possibility of cross reactivity
- ☆ Capacity building needed
- ☆ Non-specific amplification

7.12.3 Enzyme Linked Immunosorbent Assay (ELISA)

ELISA is one of the most commonly used protein based assay to detect the presence of an antibody or an antigen in a sample.

Different ELISA platforms are available for detection of antigen or antibody. The immune capture or sandwich ELISA uses capture and detecting antibodies (either specific monocolonal antibodies or polyclonal antibodies) and is used for antigen detection. The Competitive ELISA (cELISA) is an immunoassay that can be used to detect or quantify antibody/antigen using a competitive method. The cELISA for detection of specific antibodies has largely replaced the Indirect (iELISA) for large-scale screening and sero-surveillance.

Advantage

- ☆ It is a rapid, scalable, and specific assay
- ☆ Very useful for mass screening such as for animals
- ☆ The results can be measured by qualitative or quantitative means

Limitation

- ☆ Highly variable and needs skilled personnel
- ☆ It cannot differentiate between antigenically matching analytes
- ☆ Needs specific equipment such as spectrophotometric microplate reader

All the above key platforms are used for diseases diagnosis (Figure 7.7) of which ELISA was found to be common in all species except in canines wherein POC diagnostics are preferred.

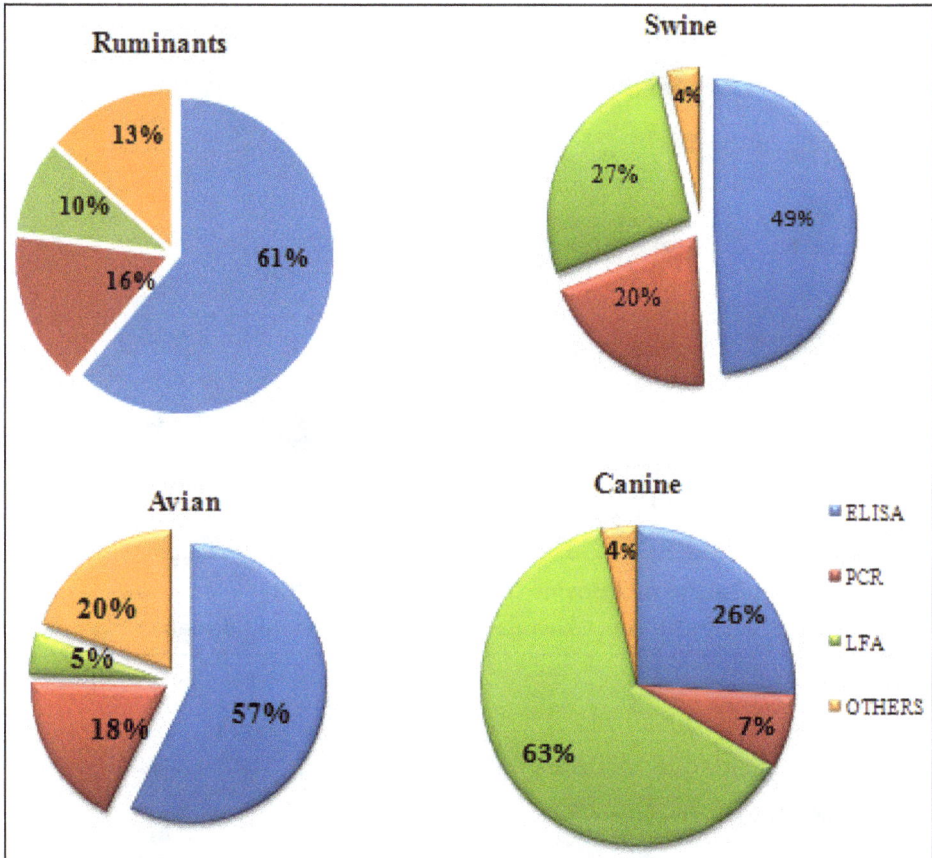

Figure 7.7: Disease Platform for Veterinary Diagnostics.

7.13 Cost of Disease Diagnostic Kits

The cost of disease diagnostic kits of bovine, avian, swine and canine were shown in Figures 7.8–7.11.

The costs of imported kits are exorbitant and hence there is an immediate need for indigenous kits with cheaper price for better applicability in clinical settings.

List of diseases for which kits are presently not available:

1. Heamorrhagic Septicaemia
2. Malignant Catarrhal Fever
3. Trypanosomiasis
4. Bovine papilloma virus
5. Avian Chlamydiosis
6. Black quarter
7. Fasciolosis
8. Pseudorabies Virus

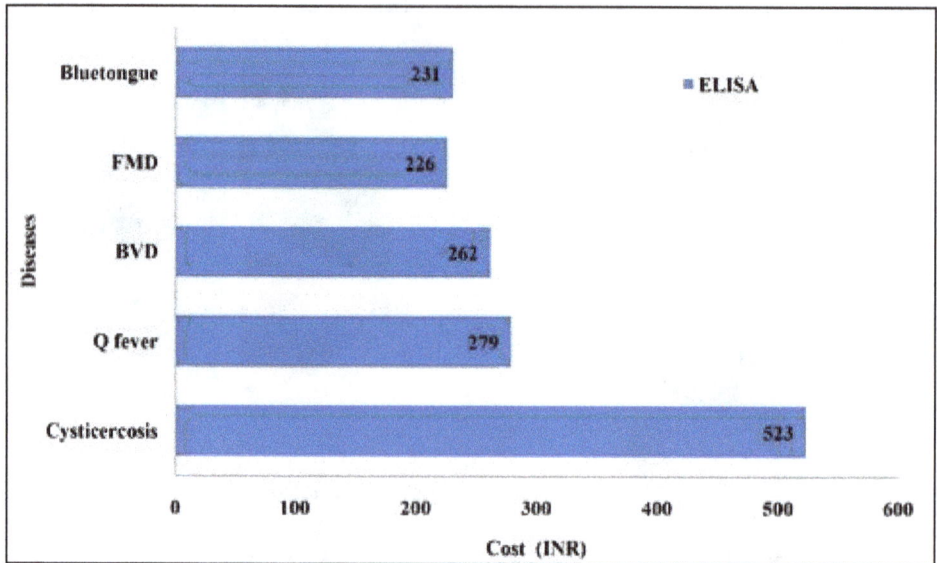

Figure 7.8: Cost of Bovine Disease Diagnostic Kit (per sample).
BVD: Bovine Viral Diarrhea; FMD: Foot and mouth disease.

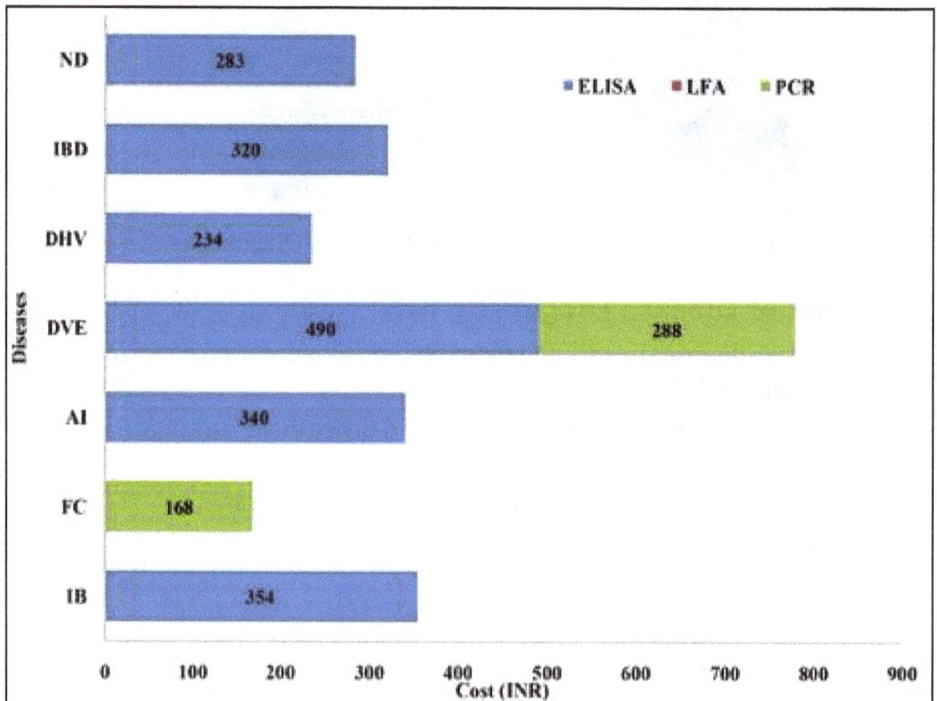

Figure 7.9: Cost of Avian Disease Diagnostic Kit (per sample).
ND: Newcastle Disease; IBD: Infectious Bursal Diseases; DHV: Duck Hepatitis Virus; DVE: Duck Virus Enteritis; AI: Avian Influenza; FC: Fowl cholera; IB: Infectious Bronchitis.

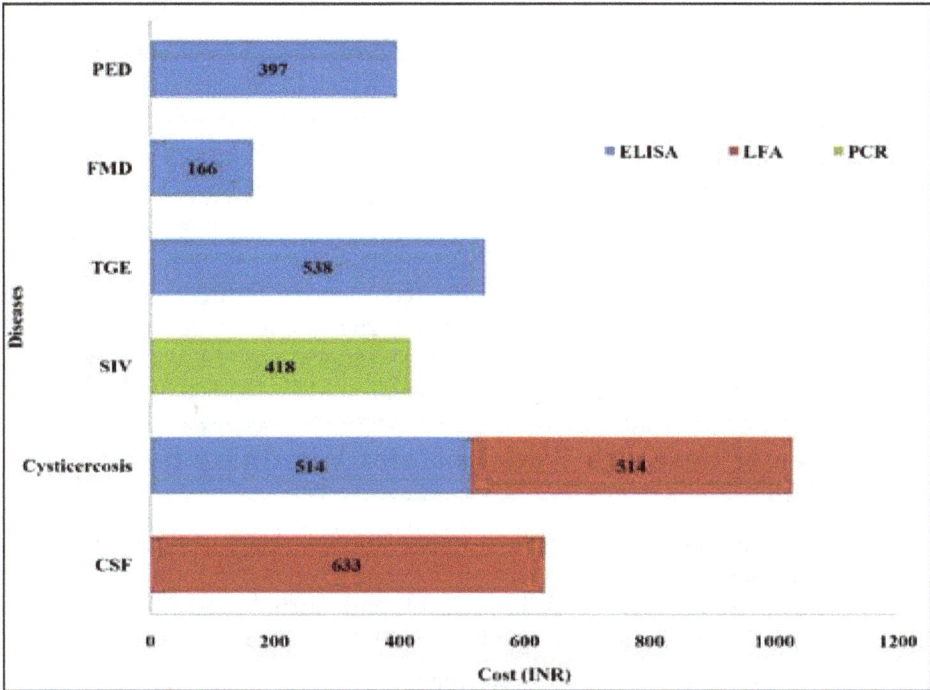

Figure 7.10: Cost of Swine Disease Diagnostic Kit (per sample).

PED: Porcine Epidemic Diarrhoea; FMD: Foot and Mouth Disease; TGE: Transmissible Gastroenteritis; SI: Swine Influenza; CSF: Classical Swine Fever.

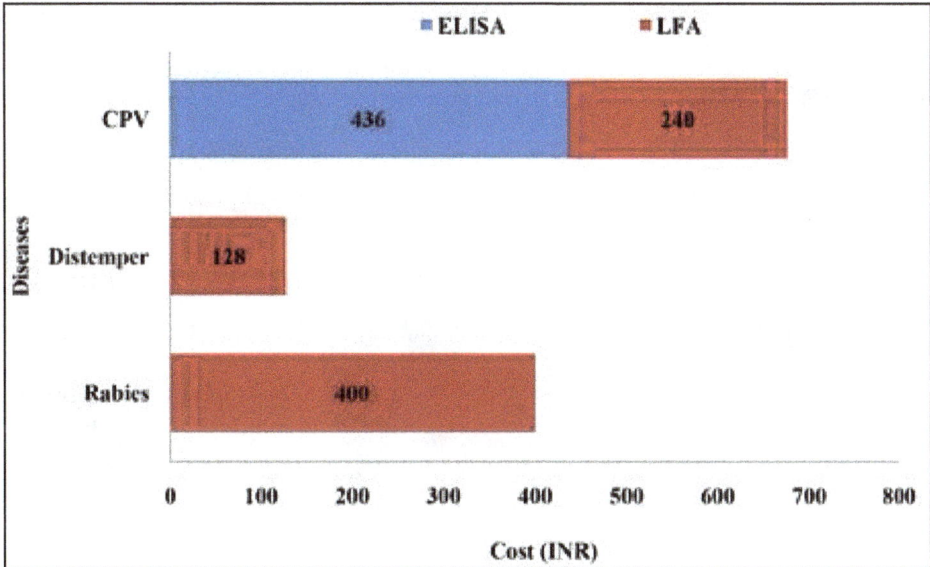

Figure 7.11: Cost of Canine Disease Diagnostic Kit (per sample).

CPV: Canine parvo virus.

Source: http://india.alibaba.com/country/products_india-veterinary-equipment.html.

☆ The ELISA based assay was commonly used for disease diagnosis in all domestic animals (Ruminants 61 per cent, avian-57 per cent, Swine-49 per cent) except canines (26 per cent) in which LFA based technology was predominantly used (63 per cent).

☆ Various diseases like Brucellosis, Bovine Viral Diarrhoea(BVD), Enzootic Bovine Leukosis (EBL), Avian Mycoplasmosis, Newcastle Disease, Transmissible Gastroenteritis (TGE) and Cysticercosis are having large number of diagnostic kits.

☆ Of the diagnostic platforms, ELISA (competitive, Indirect and sandwich) assays cost higher in the range of Rs. 250-600, followed by PCR based method with the cost ranges from Rs.160-450. The LFA kits that were used mostly in canine and swine cost around Rs.120-600.

7.14 Area of Research Work in Major Veterinary Institutes in India

☆ The analysis on major research areas of the veterinary institutes indicated that main research focus was on ruminant diseases in Indian Veterinary Research Institute (IVRI- 43 per cent) and Guru Angad Dev Veterinary and Animal Sciences University (GADVASU-48 per cent).

☆ In case of Tamil Nadu, Veterinary and Animal Sciences University (TANUVAS) the major research area is on Avian diseases (39 per cent) followed by ruminants (35 per cent) and canine disease (12 per cent). Research on canine diseases was higher at TANUVAS.

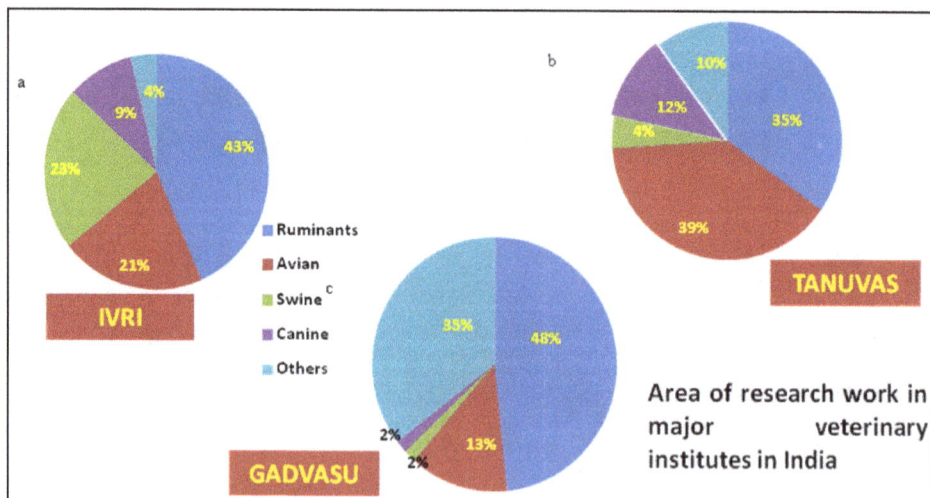

Area of research work in major veterinary institutes in India

Table 7.4: Diagnostic Kits Certified by the OIE as Validated as Fit for Purpose

Disease	Name of the Diagnostic Kit	Name of the Manufacture	Type of kit
Avian Influenza	BioChek Avian Influenza Antibody test kit	BioChek UK Ltd	ELISA
White spot disease	IQ 2000™ WSSV Detection and Prevention System	GeneReach Biotechnology Corp	PCR
Bovine spongiform encephalopathy	Prionics AG - Check Western	Prionics AG	Western Blot
Transmissible Spongiform Encephalopathies	TeSeE™ Western Blot	Bio-Rad	Western Blot
Salmonellosis Salmonella	Check and Trace	Check-Points B.V.	Multiplex LDR PCR reaction followed by detection on a diagnostic micro array
Bovine tuberculosis	*Mycobacterium bovis* Antibody Test Kit	IDEXX Laboratories	Indirect ELISA
White spot disease	IQ Plus™ WSSV Kit with POCKIT System	GeneReach Biotechnology Corp	Insulated isothermal PCR
Newcastle disease	Newcastle Disease Virus antibody detection ELISA	BioChek UK Ltd	ELISA
Bovine tuberculosis	BOVIGAM® - Mycobacterium bovis Gamma interferon test kit for cattle	Prionics AG	Sandwich ELISA

Source: OIE website (http://www.oie.int).

8

Regulations for Veterinary Biologicals

8.1 The Drugs and Cosmetics Act and Rules

The Indian pharmaceutical and drugs market is highly regulated and the regulations governing the import, manufacture, distribution and sale of drugs and cosmetics are based on the 'THE DRUGS AND COSMETICS ACT AND RULES' of Ministry of Health and Family Welfare. These regulations are implemented though Central Drugs Standard Control Organization (CDSCO) and state agencies.

As per the 'The Drugs and Cosmetics Act and Rules' "drug" include,

(i) All medicines for internal or external use of human beings or animals and all substances intended to be used for or in the diagnosis, treatment, mitigation or prevention of any disease or disorder in human beings or animals, including preparations applied on human body for the purpose of repelling insects like mosquitoes;

(ii) Such substances (other than food) intended to affect the structure or any function of the human body or intended to be used for the destruction of [vermin] or insects which cause disease in human beings or animals, as may be specified from time to time by the Central Government by notification in the Official Gazette;

The Drugs and Cosmetics Act and Rules cover both human and veterinary drugs and implemented through the same agencies (Drug Controller General of India (DCGI), CDSCO and State Government agencies).

8.2 Central Drugs Standard Control Organization (CDSCO)

CDSCO, headed by the Drug Controller General of India (DCGI) is the apex regulatory body under Ministry of Health and Family Welfare (MoHFW), Government of India. CDSCO is responsible for the approval of drugs in India. In the context of veterinary biologicals, CDSCO is responsible for grant of import/export license, clinical trial approval and new drug approvals. State Food and Drug Administration works with CDSCO in each state and is responsible for granting manufacturing license and monitoring the quality aspects of the biological, manufactured within the state. The main functions of CDSCO and State Licensing Authority is shown in Figures 8.1 and 8.2.

8.3 Regulations for Veterinary Biologics

Unlike some of the other developed countries the Drugs and Cosmetic Act, 1940 and the Drugs and Cosmetic Rules, 1945 (D and C Act and Rules) of India regulate

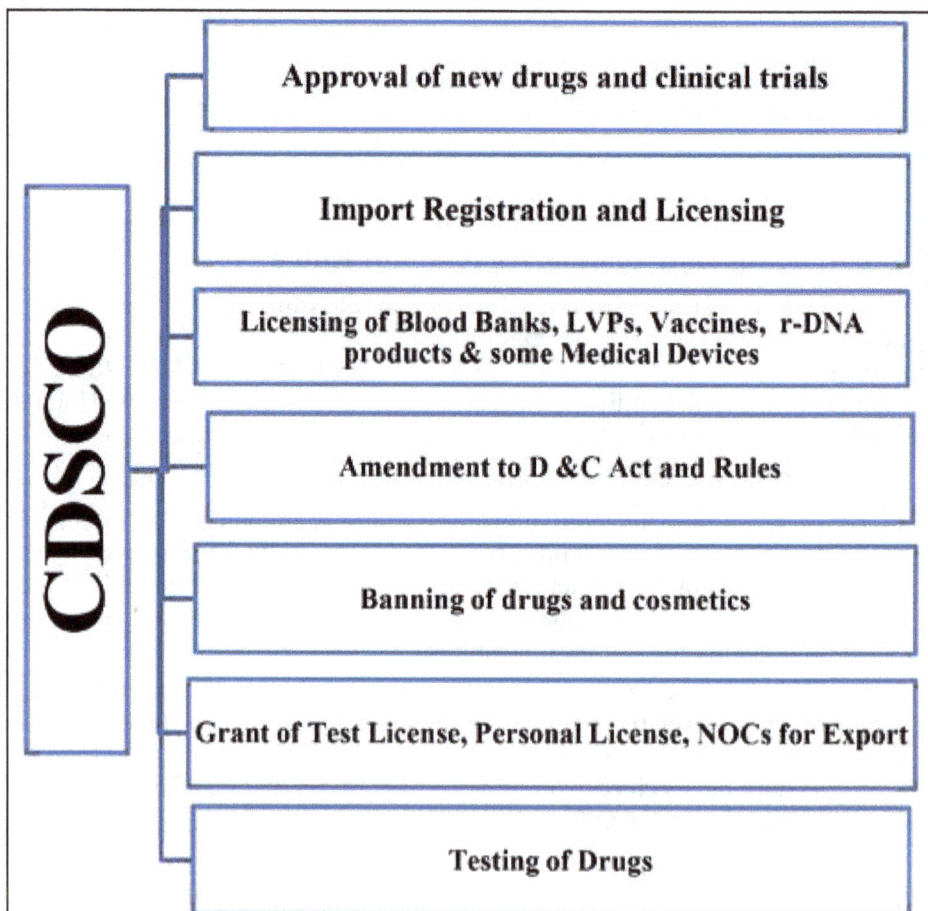

CDSCO

- Approval of new drugs and clinical trials
- Import Registration and Licensing
- Licensing of Blood Banks, LVPs, Vaccines, r-DNA products & some Medical Devices
- Amendment to D &C Act and Rules
- Banning of drugs and cosmetics
- Grant of Test License, Personal License, NOCs for Export
- Testing of Drugs

Figure 8.1: Functions of CDSCO.

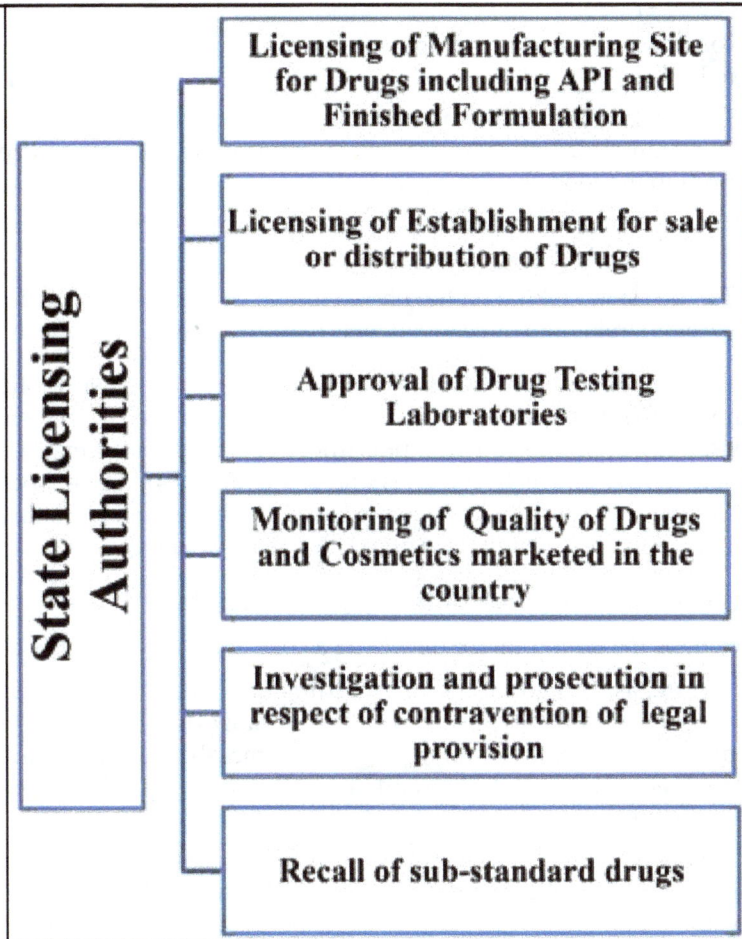

Figure 8.2: State Licensing Authorities.

both human and veterinary medicines. A separate schedule lists the production of vaccines for veterinary use (of bacterial and viral origin) and schedule F(1), part I(A) provide the requirements for bacterial vaccines and Part I(B) concerns for viral vaccines.

The regulatory requirements for veterinary biologicals/drugs differ on few counts from the human drugs.

For example,

☆ Human biologicals/new drugs require Pre-Clinical Toxicology studies (PCT) and Phase I to Phase IV clinical trials (or phase III and IV in some cases) whereas the veterinary biologicals/new drugs require a single clinical trial.

☆ Only the recombinant veterinary biologicals undergo PCT as per Review Committee on Genetic Manipulations (RCGM) recommendations and the conventional or non-recombinant veterinary biologicals are not subjected to PCT.

☆ The safety and evaluation requirements differ between the human drugs and animal drugs. Zoonotic considerations and risk assessment of the drug in the food chain are also included in the safety evaluation.

☆ Drug or biological product specific protocols are often devised to evaluate the safety and efficacy of veterinary drugs.

☆ The decision making on the import and export of veterinary biologicals, vaccine strains and infectious agents requires specific expertise in the area.

Therefore, in the case of Veterinary Medicinal Products (VMP), Ministry of Agriculture (MoA), GoI and external experts were consulted in reviewing the applications. DCGI acts, based on the inputs from Department of Animal Husbandry Dairying and Fisheries, which functions under the MoA, GoI. Some of the major decisions on the veterinary biologicals are based on the recommendations of the expert committee of Department of Animal Husbandry Dairying and Fisheries.

8.4 Regulations for New Veterinary Products

Following is the definition for new drug as per dugs and cosmetics act.

1. A drug, as defined in the Act including bulk drug substance which has not been used in the country to any significant extent under the conditions prescribed, recommended or suggested in the labelling thereof and has not been recognized as effective and safe by the licensing authority mentioned for the proposed claims.

2. A new drug already approved by the Licensing Authority for certain claims, which is now proposed to be marketed with modified or new claims, namely, indications, dosage, dosage form (including sustained release dosage form) and route of administration.

3. A fixed dose combination of two or more drugs, individually approved earlier for certain claims, which are now proposed to be combined for the first time in a fixed ratio, or if the ratio of ingredients in an already marketed combination is proposed to be changed, with certain claims, *viz.* indic ations, dosage, dosage form (including sustained release dosage form) and route of administration.

4. All vaccines shall be new drugs unless certified otherwise by the Licensing Authority

5. A new drug shall continue to be considered as new drug for a period of four years from the date of its first approval or its inclusion in the Indian Pharmacopoeia, whichever is earlier.

Therefore, any veterinary medicine, that has been marketed for less than four years in India and all the veterinary biological products will be considered as a new medicine and has to follow the procedure of a new medicine submission and approval.

The green boxes indicate recombinant products (Figure 8.3). The recombinant veterinary products undergo pre-clinical toxicity studies as per Review Committee on Genetic Manipulation (RCGM) guidelines. All the RCGM applications are routed through Institutional Biosafety Committee (IBSC).

8.5 Test Manufacturing License

Once the proof of concept is established for a veterinary biological product, test manufacturing license application in form 30 is submitted to DCGI. In response, state drug authorities visit the facility and evaluate the product, process, documents and

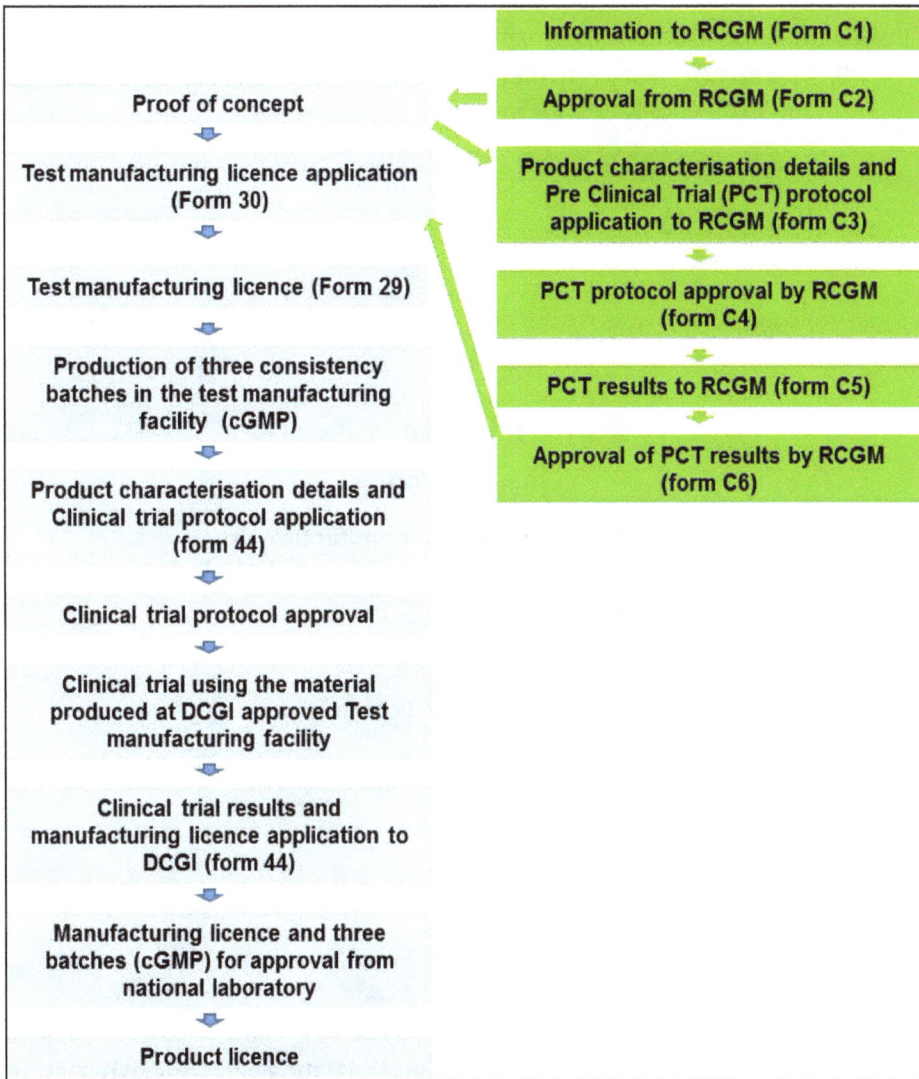

Figure 8.3: Regulatory Pathway for Veterinary Biological Products.

premises for cGMP compliance. The test manufacturing license is provided in form 29 for a particular facility to manufacture a specific drug for testing (clinical trials).

FORM 29

[See Rule 89]

Licence to manufacture drugs for purposes of examination, test or analysis

1. _____of_____is hereby licensed to manufacture the drugs specified below for purposes of examination, test or analysis at_____

2. This licence is subject to the conditions prescribed in Part VII of the Drugs and Cosmetics Rules, 1945.

3. This licence shall be in force from one year from date specified below.

   Names of Drugs: _____

   Date: _____

   Licensing Authority: _____

FORM 30

[See Rule 90]

Application for licence to manufacture drugs for purposes of examination, test or analysis

I_____of_____by occupation_____ hereby apply for licence to manufacture the drugs specified below for purposes of examination test or analysis at.................................... and I undertake to comply with the conditions applicable to the licence.

Names of Drugs: _____

Date: _____

Signature: _____

8.6 Clinical Trials

As per drugs and cosmetics act "No clinical trial for a new drug, whether for clinical investigation or any clinical experiment by any institution, shall be conducted except under, and in accordance with, the permission, in writing, of the Licensing

Authority defined in clause (b) of Rule 21. All vaccines shall be new drugs unless certified otherwise by the Licensing Authority under Rule 21".

An application in form 44 is sent to DCGI for the approval of clinical trial protocol. The clinical trial is generally conducted at three different places under the supervision of government institutions such as veterinary colleges. Clinical trials are conducted using the drug manufactured at the test manufacturing facility following the cGMP procedures. The clinical trial reports are submitted to DCGI in form 44 seeking manufacturing license. Upon successful clinical trial results, drug authorities visits the facility and evaluate the product, process, documents and premises for cGMP compliance.

Table 8.1: Regulatory Requirements and Consideration for Manufacturing of Animal Healthcare Products in India

Requirements	Considerations
Critical considerations	A pharmaceutical manufacturer, located outside India has to obtain:
	☆ Registration Certificate; (Responsibility of CDSCO)
	☆ Manufacturing License. (Responsibilities of CDSCO and State Licensing Authority) and
	☆ License for sale
Time limit for VMP license	Registration Certificate is valid for a period of 3 years.
Review time	New medicine registration approval: approx.: 12-18 months
	The process of receiving import registration can take up to 12 months.
Renewal	☆ Registration Certificate: submission 9 months before expiry
	☆ Manufacturing License: submission 6 months before expiry.
Variations	Manufacturing License: changes in the company immediately submission of new data.
	Registration certificate: variations must be classified in minor and major changes
Data protection periods for new products	Today, there is no specific law for data exclusivity in India. Indian Patents Act, 1970: Applicable only to patentable inventions, no protection for new use of a known substance or formulations by combinations. Further patent protection extends only to the invention but not to the data generated by the originator.
	The CDSCO does not provide any exclusivity for the 1st Biologic. But since all biologics are considered "New Medicines" any subsequent similar biologics need to go through the tedious process of a "New Medicine" approval.
Manufacturing license	A manufacturing license is valid for a period of 5 years.
Certificate of Pharmaceutical Product (CPP)	For import of VMPs submission of a CPP is necessary.
Labelling requirements	Not specified.
Maximum Residual Level (MRL)	For veterinary products residues, there is no specific regulation available in India

8.7 Product Licensing (Tables 8.1 and 8.2)

Product manufacturing is commenced after obtaining the manufacturing license in Form 46. Representative samples of the drug from three batches are sent to national reference laboratory for testing. For veterinary biologicals Indian Veterinary Research Institute (IVRI), Izatnagar, is the only approved national reference laboratory. Product licensing and market authorization is provided to the manufacturer after getting the clearance from national reference laboratory. Each batch of the product is released as per the specifications of Indian pharmacopeia.

Table 8.2: Regulatory Requirements and Consideration for Importing of Animal Healthcare Products in India

Requirements	Considerations
Critical considerations	A pharmaceutical manufacturer, located outside India has to obtain:
	☆ Import License; (Responsibility of CDSCO)
	☆ Registration Certificate; (Responsibility of CDSCO)
	☆ Manufacturing License. (Responsibilities of CDSCO and State Licensing Authority) and
	☆ License for sale
Review time	Import registration approval: approx.: 6-9 months;
	The process of receiving import registration can take up to 12 months.
Renewal	The following documents must be renewed regularly:
	☆ Import License: submission 3 months before expiry
	☆ Registration Certificate: submission 9 months before expiry
Variations	Import License: changes in the company immediately submission of new data.
	Registration certificate: variations must be classified in minor and major changes

FORM 44

[See rules 122A, 122B, 122D and 122 DA]

Application for grant of permission to import or manufacture a New Drug or to undertake clinical trial

I/We _____ of M/s._____(address) hereby apply for grant of permission for import and/or clinical trial or for approval to manufacture a new drug or fixed dose combination or subsequent permission for already approved new drug. The necessary information/data is given below:

1. Particulars of New Drug :

   (1) Name of the drug :

   (2) Dosage Form :

   (3) Composition of the formulation:

   (4) Test specification:

(i) Active ingredients :

(ii) Inactive ingredients :

(5) Pharmacological classification of the drug:

(6) Indications for which proposed to be used:

(7) Manufacturer of the raw material (bulk drug substances)

(8) Patent status of the drug.

2. Data submitted along with the application (as per Schedule Y with indexing and page numbers)

A. Permission to market a new drug:

(1) Chemical and Pharmaceutical information

(2) Animal Pharmacology

(3) Animal Toxicology

(4) Human/Clinical Pharmacology (Phase I)

(5) Exploratory Clinical Trials (Phase II)

(6) Confirmatory Clinical Trials (Phase III) (including published review articles)

(7) Bio-availability, dissolution and stability study Data

(8) Regulatory status in other countries

(9) Marketing information:

(a) Proposed product monograph

(b) Drafts of labels and cartons

(10) Application for test license

B. Subsequent approval/permission for manufacture of already approved new drug :

(a) Formulation:

(1) Bio-availability/bio-equivalence protocol

(2) Name of the investigator/center

(3) Source of raw material (bulk drug substances) and stability study data.

(b) Raw material (bulk drug substances)

(1) Manufacturing method

(2) Quality control parameters and/or analytical specification, stability report.

(3) Animal toxicity data.

C. Approval/Permission for fixed dose combination:
   (1) Therapeutic Justification.

   (authentic literature in peer-reviewed journals/text books)

   (2) Data on pharmacokinetics/pharmacodynamics combination.

   (3) Any other data generated by the applicant on the safety and efficacy of the combination.

D. Subsequent Approval or approval for new indication – new dosage form
   (1) Number and date of Approval/permission already granted.

   (2) Therapeutic justification for new claim/modified dosage form

   (3) Data generated on safety, efficacy and quality parameters.

A total fee of rupees_____(in words)_____has been credited to the Government under the Head of Account_____ (Photocopy of receipt is enclosed).

*Dated:*_____

Signature: _____

Designation: _____

FORM 46

[See Rules 122 B, 122 D and 122 DA]

Permission/Approval for manufacture of new drug formulation

Number of permission and date of issue _____M/s_____ _____of_____(address) is hereby granted Permission/Approval to manufacture following new drug formulation under rule 122 B/122 D/122 DA of the Drugs and Cosmetics Rules, 1945, namely :-

(1) Name of the formulation:

(2) Dosage form:

(3) Composition:

(4) Indications:

*Signature*_____

*Date:*_____

Name and designation of Licensing Authority _____

8.8 Indian Pharmacopoeia Commission

Indian Pharmacopoeia Commission (IPC) is an Autonomous Institution of the Ministry of Health and Family Welfare, Govt. of India. IPC is created to set standards for drugs in the country. It publishes official documents for improving Quality of Medicines by way of adding new and updating existing monographs in the form of Indian Pharmacopoeia (IP). IPC has 14 working groups of which one group is concerned with veterinary products.

8.9 Regulations for Recombinant Veterinary Products

The Ministry of Environment, Forests and Climate Change (MoEF&CC) has created the "Rules for the Manufacture, Use, Import, Export and Storage of Hazardous Microorganisms/Genetically Engineered Organisms or Cells, 1989 (Rules1989)" under the Environment (Protection) Act, 1986. These rules cover the area of research as well as large scale applications of GMOs and products thereof and accordingly the recombinant biological products are regulated under these rules from the research and product development stage up to its release into the environment. Various other applicable guidelines are as follows:

☆ Recombinant DNA Safety Guidelines, 1990

☆ Guidelines for generating preclinical and clinical data for rDNA vaccines, diagnostics and other biologicals, 1999

☆ CDSCO guidance for industry, 2008:
  i. Submission of Clinical Trial Application for Evaluating Safety and Efficacy
  ii. Requirements for permission of New Drugs Approval
  iii. Post approval changes in biological products: Quality, Safety and Efficacy Documents
  iv. Preparation of the Quality Information for Drug Submission for New Drug Approval: Biotechnological/Biological Products

☆ Guidelines and Handbook for Institutional Biosafety Committees (IBSCs), 2011

☆ Guidelines on Similar Biologics: Regulatory Requirements for Marketing Authorization in India, 2012

8.10 Competent Authorities

The relevant competent authorities involved in the approval process of recombinant pharmaceutical products include Institutional Biosafety Committee (IBSC), Review Committee on Genetic Manipulation (RCGM) and Genetic Engineering Appraisal Committee (GEAC).

1. Review Committee on Genetic Manipulation (RCGM)

RCGM functions in the Department of Biotechnology (DBT), Ministry of Science and Technology, Government of India. In the context of recombinant veterinary biologicals, RCGM is responsible for authorizing import/export of materials for research and development purpose; review and monitoring the recombinant drug development activities up to preclinical evaluation stage.

2. Genetic Engineering Appraisal Committee (GEAC)

GEAC functions under the Ministry of Environment and Forests (MoEF&CC) as statutory body for review and approval of activities involving large scale use of genetically engineered organisms (also referred as living modified organisms) and products thereof in research and development, industrial production, environmental release and field applications.

3. Institutional Biosafety Committee (IBSC)

IBSC functions in the concerned institution/company with the representatives from RCGM. IBSC sends its reports to RCGM. IBSC examines the applications related to r-DNA work, adherence to the *r*-DNA safety guidelines-1990, examines the containment facilities at R&D, production components and update RCGM about the facilities and makes development plan according to guidelines. IBSC provides approval for the handling of recombinant products and high risk category organisms and related experiments using these materials. All the applications to RCGM are sent with the approval of IBSC.

8.11 Licensing of Recombinant Veterinary Products

Information on initiating the research work on rDNA products and high risk category organisms are sent to RCGM through IBSC in form C1. RCGM provides its approval in form C2.

Unlike the non-recombinant veterinary biological products, the recombinant products undergo preclinical toxicology (PCT) studies as per Schedule Y of Drugs and Cosmetics Act. Application for the PCT studies is sent to RCGM in form C3. Complete product characterization details and proposed PCT protocol are included in the application. Information on preparation of Master Cell Bank and Working Cell Bank, QC test performed, techniques for the target gene expression in host cell line, complete genetic analysis like inserts, copy number and constancy, target gene expression level, production process, quality control and assurance, approved methods for the extraction and investigating the physico-chemical, biochemical, immunological and pharmacological description of the bulk, classification of the completed formulation. The IP, USP, BP or other national/international described acceptable standards for bulk and formulation, test on efficacy of the target product, data related to batch fermentation of the product, impurity valuation like DNA, RNA, lipids, carbohydrates, proteins from the host organisms and any toxic material in the product.

RCGM provides its approval for PCT protocol in form C4. The applicant performs the PCT studies as per the approved protocol. PCT studies of veterinary biological products are performed in target species in contrast to the human products (PCT studies of human products are performed in laboratory animals). PCT study results are provided by the applicant to RCGM in form C5. In response, RCGM recommends DCGI for considering the product for the clinical trials. The clinical trials are performed as per the procedure described earlier.

If the product contains any live recombinant organism, additional risk assessment is performed by GEAC before conducting the clinical trials. GEAC assesses the impact of the recombinant organism on environment during the large scale production of the product and application of the product in the animals/humans.

Form C1

Information to RCGM to carryout research involving genetically modified organisms (GMOs)/living modified organisms (LMOs) for development of rDNA products for healthcare and industria use

1. Name of the Applicant:

    Designation:

    Address:

    Telephone No.:   Fax No.:   e-mail:

2. DBT Office Memorandum No.:

3. **Application for :**

    3.1 Purpose: (not more than 100 words)
        1. New Ongoing Project
            If yes, No. and Date of permission letter issued :
            Yes   No
        2. Category (Biosafety level) of experiments as per the Recombinant DNA safety Guidelines, 1990 issued by DBT

4. **Description of the GMOs/LMOs proposed to employed in the research proposal:**

    (in scientific terms; for new application only)

    4.1 Description of GMOs/LMOs

    4.2 Description of the target gene(s)

    4.3 Number of copies of the genes incorporated

    4.4 Description of the target product(s)

5. **Details on :**

    5.1 Source of nucleic acid(s) :

    5.2 Nucleic acid sequence (Please enclose the nucleic acid sequence map of the target gene) :

    5.3 Vector(s) (Please enclose the map of the vector gene) :

    5.4 Host(s) that carrying the vector(s)/target gene(s) :

5.5 Manipulative procedures:

5.6 Anticipated functions of product(s)

6. **Summary of the proposed work plan utilizing GMOs:**

(please check it from the following areas and provide the details of work plan).

6.1 Basic transformation and laboratory work to assess the expression of the target gene

6.2 Standardization of fermentation/production procedures

7. **Site/Location of the research work :**

8. **Proposed containment facility (Please indicate the level of containment proposed):**

9. **Decontamination and disposal mechanisms:**

10. **Risk management (Emergency plan):**

11. Any other relevant information:

12. Declaration :

I declare that the information provided in the given format is correct and accurate to the best of my knowledge. The Safety Guidelines brought out by the Department of Biotechnology, Ministry of Science and Technology, Govt. of India will be and is being strictly followed. In case any untoward incident occurs, the Chairman of the IBSC and the Member Secretary of the RCGM will be informed immediately.

Date: *Signature of the Applicant* _____

Forwarded:

The proposal set out above has been considered and approved by the Institutional Biosafety Committee in its meeting held on and is forwarded to RCGM for further necessary action.

Date: *Signature and name of the Chairman, IBSC*

Note:

1. Please submit 23 copies of the application along with the enclosures to the Mem ber Secretary, RCGM, Department of Biotechnology for consideration by RCGM.

2. Enclosed: (Kindly tick the enclosures)

   a. Sequence map of the gene

   b. Vector Map

   c. Copy of the permit, if issued earlier

   d. Copy of the minutes of IBSC meeting in which the proposal was approved

Form C2

Informtaion on record take by RCGM for research involving genetically modified organisms (GMOs)/living modified organisms (LMOs) for development of rDNA products for healthcare and industrial use

PERMIT NUMBER: **DATE OF ISSUE:**

DATE OF EXPIRY:

Applicant:

Name of Organisation:

Address:

Phone, fax and e.mail:

Subject: Information submitted vide letter No.   **Dated**

1. This is to inform that the application to Review Committee on Genetic Manipulation (RCGM) on the following projects was considered and noted by the RCGM in its meeting held on_____.

   i)

   ii)

2. Additional information sought by RCGM, if any should be separately included.

3. You are required to comply with the rDNA Safety Guidelines1990 of DBT.

4. Please provide the information on the above projects for updation on http://www.igmoris.nic.in as per details on the website

(Member Secretary, RCGM)

Form C3

Application to RCGM to conduct preclinical and/or safety studies of rDNA products developed using genetically modified organisms (GMOs)/living modified organisms (LMOs) for healthcare, industrial or any other use

1. **Name of the Applicant:**

   Designation:

   Address:

   Telephone No.:   Fax No.:   email:

2. **DBT Office Memorandum No.:**

3. **Application for :**

   3.1 Purpose (not more than 100 words)

   3.2 New   Yes   No

   3.3 Ongoing Project   Yes   No

   If yes, No. and Date of permission letter issued and also briefly state the purpose for which permission was granted.

   3.4 Category (Biosafety level) of experiments as per the Guidelines of DBT

4. **Objectives of the proposal:**

5. **Background about the nature of the product with appropriate references:**

   (may include in about 100 words, the process of development, mode of action, thera peutic indication, therapeutic dose if available, whether product is already in use elsewhere, if yes, any known side effects, animal toxicology data, similarity/dissimi larity between the molecule/compound under consideration)

6. **Molecular biology details of the GMOs/LMOs employed:**

   6.1 Origin of gene

   6.2 Sequence

   6.3 Vector/promoter/terminator

   6.4 Transformation process

   6.5 Host organism characteristics

   6.6 Safety of the organism

   6.7 Copy number of the plasmid

   6.8 Stability data of the plasmid

   6.9 Expression level in the host

   6.10 Containment levels and biosafety

7. Standardization of fermentation/production procedures:

7.1 Basic transformation and laboratory work to assess the expression of the target gene.

7.2 Five batches of reproducible fermentation data (Batch size adequate to give after purification enough purified product to generate preclinical data) with detail kinetics of one single batch.

7.3 Fermentation kinetics data from one representative batch indicating cell growth, product formation, pH, temperature, dissolved oxygen, major nutri ent consumption pattern, RPM for agitation.

7.4 Concentration of product/L, yield and volumetric productivity.

(Provide details to show that the specific protein yield (amount of protein per unit cell mass) remains more or less constant at different cell concentration during fermentation).

8. Downstream process for purification:

8.1 Steps involved in purification of the product

8.2 Batch size for protein purification

8.3 Description of each unit operation step during purification and recovery of protein

8.4 Quality of the product and recovery efficiency

8.5 Overall recovery of the product in each batch operation

8.6 Consistency of recovery in 5 consecutive batches of purification

9. Product/protein characterization:

9.1 Molecular weight/western blot/SDSPAGE/mass spec

9.2 Amino acid sequence (10 N terminal AA)

9.3 Peptic digest

9.4 Secondary structure by CD (near and far UV)

9.5 Fluorescence spectra

9.6 Disulfide bond presence if any

9.7 Carbohydrate content and details of components (for glycoproteins)

9.8 Presence of aggregates

9.9 Host cell protein/contaminants

9.10 Residual DNA and LPS/endotoxin

9.11 Pyrogen content

10. Formulation and stability studies:

10.1 Extended stability

10.2 Use of stabilizer(s) and its concentration

10.3 Product quality in formulated condition

10.4 Bioactivity/immunogenicity of the formulated product

11. Efficacy of the product: Information on:

  11.1 Receptor binding assay if any

  11.2 Cellular proliferation assay

  11.3 Signal transduction pathways

  11.4 Tissue specific a ctivity

  11.5 *In vivo* studies in animal models

  11.6 Pharmacokinetics and Pharmacodynamics studies

12. Immunogenicity studies:

  12.1 equence specific

  12.2 Non Specific to other proteins

  12.3 Immunogenicity with adjuvants

13. Acceptability criteria of the bulk and the formulated material wherever ready for preclinical or safety studies:

14. Proposed work plan for preclinical or other safety studies:

  14.1 List of the studies to be done

  14.2 Information about the route of administration, dose, vehicle, mode of administration in each study

  14.3 Basis of dose calculation for each animal used (indicate the guidelines followed such as ScheduleY, ICH, FDA or justify deviations if any).

  14.4 Toxicity and allergenicity protocols

  (Provide complete study design including test species, age, body weight, control groups such as vehicle control, comparator group, recovery groups, details of biochemical, histopathological and other parameters to be mea sured, organs to be weight, monitoring schedule *etc.*)

  14.5 Address and accreditation status of the labs where studies proposed to be conducted.

  14.6 Status of Institutional Animal Ethics Committee.s Approval (Please specify the studie and products to be tested in each lab).

15. Proposed containment facility as well as measures:

16. Decontamination and disposal mechanisms:

17. Risk management (Emergency plan):

18. Any other relevant information:

19. Declaration :

  I declare that the information provided in the above format is correct and accurate to the best of my knowledge. The Safety Guidelines brought out by the Department of Biotechnology, Ministry of Science and Technology, Govt. of India will be and is being strictly followed. In case any untoward incident occurs, the Chairman of the IBSC and the MemberSecretary of the RCGM will be informed immediately.

Date: *Signature of the Applicant* _____

Forwarded:

The proposal set out above has been considered and approved by the Institutional Biosafety Committee in its meeting held on and is forwarded to RCGM for further necessary action.

Date: *Signature and name of the Chairman, IBSC*

Note:

1. Please submit 23 copies of the application along with the enclosures to the Member Secretary, RCGM, Department of Biotechnology for consideration by RCGM.

2. Enclosed: (Kindly tick the enclosures):
    ☆ Sequence map of the gene
    ☆ Vector Map
    ☆ Copy of the import/receive permits, or any other approval letters issued earlier
    ☆ Copy of the minutes of IBSC meeting in which the proposal was approved

Form C4

Permit for conduct of preclinical safety studies of rDNA product(s) in healthcare

PERMIT NUMBER: **DATE OF ISSUE:**

DATE OF EXPIRY:

Permittee:

Name of Organisation:

Address:

Phone, fax and email:

Subject:

AUTHORISATION:

This is in response to your letter no. _____dated_____on the above mentioned subject.   It is informed that your application was considered by the Review Committee on Genetic Manipulation (RCGM) in its meeting held on. On the basis of the recommendations of the RCGM and comments of the experts on the dossier, you are allowed to conduct preclinical safety studies onon the premises located at subject to the acceptance of the following terms and conditions:

A. There would be no change in the protocols approved by RCGM which includes :

1. You would follow the protocols as per the Schedule "Y" of the Drugs and Cosmetics Act of 1940 and Rules 1945 of the Govt of India.

2. The route of administration of the product in lab animals would be the same as of therapeutic route of administration and any other route specified in the protocols.

3. You would conduct laboratory studies with proper controls and reference mate rials.

4. You are also directed to include a control group of animals by taking innovators product as gold standard in toxicity studies for comparison as per the Schedule Y of the Drugs and Cosmetics Act of 1940 and Rules1945 of the Govt. of India.

5. You would be using the protocols in terms of dose fixation as was submitted to the RCGM Secretariat.

6. You would use the formulated material of in these studies as far as equivalent to the final product to be used commercially at later stage. You would maintain sufficient stocks of the formulated materials as reference inventory in proper storage conditions with the batch details of such stocks, which would be pro vided by you to the Competent Authority before starting the experiments as well as after completion of the studies. There would not be any subsequent ma jor modifications or changes in the composition of the formulated material utilized in toxicology studies in animals after finalization of studies. In case of any subsequent change, the production methods or the quality of the bulk as well as the formulated material, it is to be brought to the notice of the Competent Authority and no such altered materials be used by you for commercial purpose or other wise without prior approval from the Statutory and Competent Authority.

7. You would ascertain and maintain that only organisations authorized personnel would be allowed to visit the experimental lab and the details of personnel visiting the lab. with dates, purpose(s) *etc.* would be maintained in register, which may be available for inspection, whenever required by the Competent Authority.

8. You would inform the RCGM through your Institutional Biosafety Committee (IBSC) the progress of work from time to time. The IBSC will collect all the infor mation on experiments and would submit the consolidated information/data/results on experiments to the RCGM once in a year.

9. You would adhere to the Recombinant DNA Safety Guidelines, 1990 and also follow the other Guidelines for generating preclinical and clinical data for *r*DNA based vaccines, diagnostics and other biologicals brought out by the Department of Biotechnology, the Government of India, from time to time. Accidents, if any, arising out of the experiments would be brought to the notice of the Govt. immediately.

10. You are required to confirm the acceptance of the above conditions to the DBT at your earliest convenience before starting the toxicity studies. You are further informed that you may contact the Department of Biotechnology for any clarifi cation in the matter, which you may require.

PERIOD: The permit letter shall be in force from to unless it is sooner suspended or cancelled under the said Rules.

Kindly acknowledge the receipt of the same

(Member Secretary, RCGM)

Copy for information to:

1. The Chairman, GEAC, Ministry of Environment, Forest and Climate Change, Indira Paryavaran Bhavan, Jorbagh Road, New Delhi - 110 003

2. The Secretary, Ministry of Health and Family Welfare, Nirman Bhawan, New Delhi 1.

3. The Drugs Controller General of India, FDA Bhawan, Kotla Road, New Delhi 110 002.

4. The Director General, Indian Council of Medical Research, Ansari Nagar, Post Box No.4911, New Delhi 110 029.

5. Office copy for file

6. Guard File

Form C5

Format for submission of preclinical or other safety studies report of rDNA products developed using genetically modified organisms (GMOs)/ living modified organisms (LMOs) for healthre, industrial or any other use

1. **Name of the Applicant:**

    Designation:

    Address:

    Telephone No.: Fax No.: email:

2. **DBT Office Memorandum No.:**

3. **Objectives of the proposal:**

4. **Summary of the products characteristics and process of development:**

5. **List of preclinical study protocols approved by RCGM:**
    (*please attach a copy of the approval letter*)

6. **Preclinical study reports:**

    6.1 List of studies completed and deviations, if any from the approved protocols

    6.2 Dose calculation for conduct of safety studies

    6.3 Study reports (Each study report would reflect all the issues approved in the protocols). In addition the following to be included:

    RCGM approval of protocol

    IBSC approval of report

    6.4 IAEC approval for animal use and for the procedures

    ☆ Individual animal data, summary data and any other data like computer analysis outputs etc

    ☆ Conclusion

    6.4 Address and accreditation status of the labs where these studies were con ducted.

7. **Measures taken for containment:**

8. **Decontamination and disposal mechanisms:**

9. **Risk management (Emergency plan):**

10. **Any other relevant information:**

11. Declaration:

I declare that the information provided in the above format is correct and accurate to the best of my knowledge.

Date: *Signature of the Applicant* _____

Forwarded:

The proposal set out above has been considered and approved by the Institutional Biosafety Committee in its meeting held on and is forwarded to RCGM for further necessary action.

Date: **Signature and name of the Chairman, IBSC**

Note:

1. Please submit 23 copies of the application along with the enclosures to the Member Secretary, RCGM, Department of Biotechnology for consideration by RCGM.

2. Enclosures should include

   a. Copies of earlier approvals from RCGM

   b. Copy of the minutes of IBSC meeting in which the proposal was approved

Form C6

Recommendation of rDNA product(s) for healthcare use to DCG(I) for the appropriate phase of clinical trial

PERMIT NUMBER: **DATE OF ISSUE:**

To

The Drug Controller General of India,

C.H.E.B.Campus, FDA Bhawan,

Kotla Road, New Delhi 110 002.

Subject:

M/s._____, was granted permission vide letter no. dated to conduct preclinical safety studies in the premises located at_____

It is informed that reports on pre clinical safety studies on_____

Based on the submissions made by the applicant and the recommendations of the RCGM, the applicant has been directed to approach your office for approval to conduct appropriate Phase of human clinical trials on

by submitting all relevant information.

Kindly acknowledge the receipt of the same

Member Secretary, RCGM)

Copy for information to:

1. The Chairman, GEAC, Ministry of Environment and Forests, Paryavaran Bhawan, CGO Complex, Lodi Road, New Delhi 110 003

2. M/s_____(applicant)

3. Office copy for file

4. Guard file

8.12 Import of Veterinary Biologicals for Research Purpose Including Clinical Trials

An application for a licence for examination, test or analysis shall be made in Form 12 and shall be made or countersigned by the head of the institution in which, or by a proprietor or director or the company or firm by which the examination, test or analysis will be conducted.

In response DCGI issues import permit in form 11. DCGI seeks the advice of ministry of agriculture wherever it is necessary. For conducting clinical trials with the imported drugs, an application in form 44 is to be submitted to DCGI.

Form 12

[*See* Rule 34]

Application for licence to import drugs for purpose of examination, test or analysis

I_____resident of_____by occupation _____hereby apply for a licence to import the drugs specified below for the purposes of examination, test or analysis at_____ from_____and I undertake to comply with the conditions applicable to the licence.

1[A fee of rupees_____has been credited to Government under the head of Account '0210-Medical and Public Health, 04-Public Health, 104-Fees and Fines under the Drugs and Cosmetics Rules, 1945—Central vide Challan No_____dated_____(attached in original).]

Names of drugs and classes of drugs Quantities _____

Date: _____

Signature: _____

Form 11

[*See* Rule 33]

Licence to import drugs for the purposes of examination, test or analysis

1. I_____of_____is hereby licensed to import from _____the drugs specified below for the purposes of examination, test or analysis at_____or in such other places as the licensing authority may from time to time authorize.

2. This licence is subject to the conditions prescribed in the Rule under the Drugs and Cosmetics Act, 1940.

3. This licence shall, unless previously suspended or revoked, be in force for a period of one year from the date specified below_____

Names of drugs: _____ *Quantity which may be imported*

Date: _____

Licensing Authority: _____

8.13 Import of Recombinant Materials for Research Purpose

For the import of recombinant materials for research purpose, an application to RCGM is submitted in form **B1** through IBSC.

Form B1

Appication to RCGM for import of genetically modified orgnasisms (GMOs)/living modified organisms (LMOs) and product(s) thereore for research and development purpose

1. **Name of the Applicant:**

   Designation: Contact Address:

   Telephone No: Fax No: email:

2. DBT Office Memorandum No.:

3. Objectives of the proposal:

4. Description of the GMOs/LMOs and product thereof (in scientific terms):

  (a) Morphology

  (b) Physiology

  (c) Pathogenicity, if any

  (d) Number of copies of the genes incorporated

  (e) Status of approval is country of origin.

5. Details on:

  (a) Source of nucleic acid(s):

  (b) Nucleic acid sequence (Please enclose the nucleic acid sequence map of the target gene):

  (c) Vector(s) (Please enclose the map of the vector):

  (d) Sequence of the genes incorporated/to be incorporated into the host organism.

  (e) Host(s) carrying the vector(s)/target gene(s):

  (f) Manipulative procedures used:

6. Quantity of GMOs/LMOs and products thereof to be imported:

(Please specify the number and type of total packs such as vials, plates *etc.* and the size/quantity in each pack)

7. Details of earlier imports:

  7.1 Whether the proposed GMOs/LMOs and products thereof was imported earlier:

  Yes   No

  If yes, provide the copy of relevant permit issued previously and quanities imported (please specify the number of total packs such as vials, plates *etc.* and the size in each pack and the total quantity as the case may be).

  7.2 Statement of utilization on the earlier GMOs/LMOs and products thereof imported:

8. Proposed work plan

  8.1 Summary of the proposed work plan utilizing GMOs/LMOs and products there of: (This should indicate schematic lab work, green house or any other studies proposed to be undertaken)

  8.2 Category (biosafety level) of experiments to be done as per the Recombinant _ DNA Safety Guidelines issued by DBT:

9. Source and transport details:

9.1 Source of GMOs/LMOs and products thereof proposed to be imported:

Name of the Agency: _____

Contact person: _____

Address: _____

Telephone No.: _____

Fax No.: _____

Email: _____

9.2 Mode of Transport:

Rail   Road   Air   Ship

9.3 Safety norms to be observed during transit:

10. Proposed containment facility:

(Please indicate the level of containment proposed)

11. Proposed decontamination, disposal mechanisms and risk management measures:

12. Any other relevant information:

13. Declaration:

I declare that the information provided in the above format is correct and accurate to the best of my knowledge. The Recombinant DNA Safety Guidelines issued by the Department of Biotechnology, Ministry of Science and Technology, Govt. of India will be strictly followed. The imported material will be utilized for the said purpose only. In case any untoward incident occurs, the Chairman of the IBSC and the Member Secretary of the RCGM will be informed immediately.

*Date:*_____   *Signature of the Applicant* _____

Forwarded: _____

The proposal set out above has been considered and approved by the nstitutional Biosafety Committee on its meeting held on and is forwarded to RCGM for further necessary action.(copy of the minutes of relevant meeting en closed)

*Date :*_____ *Signature and Name of the Chairman, IBSC*

Note: _____

1. Please submit 23 copies of the application along with the enclosures to the Member Secretary, RCGM, Department of Biotechnology for consideration by RCGM

2. Enclosures should include

    ☆ Sequence map of the gene

    ☆ Vector Map

    ☆ Copy of the import permit, if issued earlier

    ☆ Copy of the Utilization certificate, if imported earlier

    ☆ Copy of the minutes of IBSC meeting in which the proposal was approved

    ☆ Copy of the Material Transfer Agreement duly signed by both parties

8.14 Import of Drugs for Distribution or Marketing in India

Registration of the drug and the manufacturing premises is mandatory for importing any drugs into India. Application for issue of Registration Certification for import of drugs into India is made in form 40 to DCGI. The registration certificate is provided by DCGI in form 41. Apart from this an application in form 9 is to be sent by the importer for getting the import permit and in response an import permit is issued in form 10.

Form 40

[*See* rule 24-A]

Application for issue of Registration Certification for import of drugs into India under the

Drugs and Cosmetics Rules 1945.

I/We_____(Name and full address) hereby apply for the grant of Registration Certificate for the manufacturer, M/s._____(full address with telephone, fax and E-mail address of the foreign manufacturer) for his premises, and manufactured drugs meant for import into India.

1. Names of drugs for registration.

    (1)

    (2)

    (3)

    2. I/We enclose herewith the information and undertakings specified in Schedule D (1) and Schedule D (II) duly signed by the manufacturer for grant of Registration Certificate for the premises stated below.

    3. A fee of_____for registration of premises, the particulars of which are given below, of the manufacturer has been credited to the Government under the Head of Account "0210-Medical and Public Health,

04-Public Health, 104-Fees and Fines under Drugs and Cosmetics Rules, 1945 – Central vide Challan No._____dated, (attached in original).

4. A fee of_____for registration of the drugs for import as specified at Serial No.2 above has been credited to the Government under the Head of Account "0210-Medical and Public Health, 04-Public Health, 104- Fees and Fines" under the Drugs and Cosmetics Rules, 1945 – Central vide Challan No._____, dated_____. (attached original).

5. Particulars of premises to be registered where manufacture is carried on:

Address (es) _____

Telephone No. _____

Fax _____

E-mail _____

I/We undertake to comply with all terms and conditions required to obtain Registration Certificate and to keep it valid during its validity period.

PLACE

DATE

*Signature*_____
*Name*_____
*Designation*_____

Seal/Stamp of manufacturer or his authorized agent in India

Form No. 41

[See rule 27-A]

Registration Certificate

Registration Certificate to be issued for import of drugs into India under Drugs and Cosmetics Rules, 1945

Registration Certificate No._____Date_____
M/s_____(Name and full address of registered office)_____
having factory premises at_____(full address) has been registered

under rule 27-A as a manufacturer and is hereby issued this Registration Certificate.

1. Name (s) of drugs which many be imported under this Registration Certificate:

   (1)

   (2)

   (3)

3. This Registration Certificate shall be in force from_____to _____unless it is sooner suspended or cancelled under the rules.

4. This Registration Certificate is issued through the office of the manufacturer or his authorized agent in India M/s_____(name and full address) who will be responsible for the business activities of the manufacturer, in India in all respects.

5. This Registration Certificate is subject to the conditions, stated below and to such other conditions as may be specified in the Act and the rules, from time to time.

*Place:*_____

*Date:*_____   *LICENSING AUTHORITY*

                                                          Seal/Stamp

Form 9

[*See* Rule 24]

Form of undertaking to accompany an application for an import licence

Whereas_____of_____intends to apply for a licence under the Drugs and Cosmetics Rules, 1945, for the import into India, of the drugs specified below manufactured by us, we_____of_____ hereby give this undertaking that for the duration of the said licence:

(1) the said applicant shall be our agent for the import of drugs into India;

(2) we shall comply with the conditions imposed on a licence by 1[Rules 74 and 78]of the Drugs and Cosmetics Rules, 1945;

(3) we declare that we are carrying on the manufacture of the drugs mentioned in this undertaking at the premises specified below, and we shall from time to time report any change of premises on which manufacture will be carried on and in cases where manufacture is carried on in more than one factory any change in the distribution of functions between the factories;

(4) we shall comply with the provisions of Part IX of the Drugs and Cosmetics Rules, 1945;

(5) every drug, manufactured by us for import under licence into India shall as regards strength, quality and purity conform with the provisions of Chapter III of the Drugs and Cosmetics Act, 1940, and the Drugs and Cosmetics Rules, 1945;

(6) we shall comply with such further requirements, if any, as may be specified by Rules, by the Central Government under the Act and of which the licensing authority has given to the licensee not less than four months' notice.

Names of drugs and classes of drugs _____

Particulars of premises where manufacture is carried on.

Date.............

[Signature, Name, Designation Seal/Stamp
of manufacturer or on behalf of the manufacturer]

Form 10

[See rules 23 and 27]

License to import drugs (excluding hose specified in Schedule X) to the Drugs and

Cosmetic Rules, 1945.

1. License Number_____Date _____(Name and full address of the Importer) is hereby licensed to import into India during the period for which the licence is in force, the drugs specified below, manufactured by M/s._____(name and full address) and any other drugs manufactured the said manufacturer as may from time to time be endorsed on this licence.

2. This licence shall be valid in force from_____to_____ unless it is sooner suspended or cancelled under the said rules.

3. Names of drugs to be imported.

   Place :

Date:_____

LICENSING AUTHORITY

Seal/Stamp

* *Delete whichever is not applicable.*

Conditions of Licence

1. A photocopy of licence shall be displayed in a prominent place in a part of the premises, and the original licence shall be produced, whenever required.

2. Each batch of drug imported into India shall be accompanied with a detailed batch test report and a batch release certificate, duly signed and authenticated by the manufacturer with date of testing, date of release and the date of forwarding such reports. The imported batch of each drug shall be subjected to examination and testing as the licensing authority deems fit prior to its marketing.

3. The licensee shall be responsible for the business activities of the manufacturer in India along with the registration holder and his authorized agent.

4. The licensee shall inform the licensing authority forthwith in writing in the event of any change in the constitution of the firm operating under the licence. Where any change in the constitution of the firm takes place, the current license shall be deemed to be valid for a maximum period of three months from the date on which the change takes place unless, in the meantime, a fresh licence has been taken from the licensing authority in the name of the firm with the changed constitution.

8.15 CPCSEA (Committee for the Purpose of Control and Supervision on Experiments on Animals) Guidelines for Laboratory Animal Facility

The CPCSEA (Committee for the Purpose of Control and Supervision on Experiments on Animals) guidelines are regulating the laboratory experiments on animals. In these guidelines each and every point are given which are related with all laboratory animals safety and security.

The goal of these Guidelines is to promote the human care of animals used in biomedical and behavioral research and testing with the basic objective of providing specifications that will enhance animal well-being, quality in the pursuit of advancement of biological knowledge that is relevant to humans and animals. Some main points are given below from CPCSEA guidelines.

☆ Veterinary care

☆ Animal procurement

☆ Quarantine, stabilization and separation

☆ Surveillance, diagnosis, treatment and control of disease

☆ Animal care and technical personnel

☆ Personal hygiene

☆ Animal experimentation involving hazardous agents

☆ Multiple surgical procedures on single animal

☆ Durations of experiments *etc.*

For detailed information on CPCSEA guidelines visit (icmr.nic.in/bioethics/final_cpcsea.pdf)

8.16 Animal Experimentation Guidelines in India

Animals in research experiment and instruction are structured by Appendix IV of the Prevention of Cruelty to Animals Act, 1960 (PCA Act) and related Breeding and Experiments on Animals (Control and Supervision) Rules, 1998 (as amended in 2001 and 2006). The PCA act authorizes the Committee for Purpose of Control and Supervision of Experiments on Animals (CPCSEA), a legal body formed under the PCA Act, to impose the law with respect to the guideline of animal experimentation in India and use the regulation of the practice of animals in trialing, including toxicity testing:

1. Whichever institution that practices animals for research, safety testing need register itself with the CPCSEA.

2. Each institution has to custom an Institutional Animal Ethics Committee (IAEC).

3. It is accountable for examining the concerned institution's animal house and appreciative or refusing animal research projects.

4. An amendment by IAEC, brought around the Breeding of and Experiments on Animals Rules in 2006, was specified power to license only trials on small animals.

5. The central commission of the CPCSEA has the authority to support large animal experiments.

6. It has the authority to ban any kind of research upon getting a protest against an institution.

The IAEC is required to have 8 members, as follows: a biological scientist, two scientists from different biological disciplines, a veterinarian involved in the care of animal, Scientist in charge of the animal facility of the establishment concerned, a scientist from outside the institute, a non-scientific socially aware member and a nominee of CPCSEA

It is mandatory for IAEC to monitor the examination during the project and after completion of it over reports. It is compulsory to duty call the animal house and research laboratory where the experiments are lead to certify amenability with all controlling requirements, strategies and rules.

Experimentation on laboratory animals are approved by the IAEC after examining the application. Experimentation on large animals are referred to CPCSEA through IAEC and the central committee decides on the appropriateness of the large animal experimentations.

9

Biosafety

9.1 Introduction

Biosafety

As per the definition of World Health Organization (WHO), biosafety includes the containment principles, technologies and practices that are implemented to prevent unintentional exposure to pathogens and toxins, or their accidental release. Therefore, biosafety is preventing the harmful organisms from escaping from the laboratory and protecting the handlers and environment from the organisms.

Biosecurity

Biosecurity means 'protecting the pathogens from misuse, theft or intentional release' by means of proper institutional and personal security measures and procedures.

In spite of the known hazards of pathogenic micro-organisms, laboratory handling of the pathogens is often necessary:

☆ To identify the disease causing agent

☆ To develop prevention and therapeutic measures against the infectious disease

☆ To get insight into the properties of the organisms

However, personnel and environmental safety should be given the highest importance while using the pathogenic organisms for the above said reasons. Containment facilities and biocontainment-practices are therefore developed to protect laboratory personnel, adjacent communities, animal agriculture and the environment from being exposed to potentially hazardous biological agents. The choice of appropriate containment facility with the requisite infrastructure and biosafety practices depends on the risk perception levels.

9.2 Risk Perception and Biosafety Level Category of the Pathogens

Infectious agents are categorized based on their relative risk perception and the following factors are considered in making this classification.

Pathogenicity of the Organism

☆ Prevalence of the organism in a country and host range of the organism

☆ Mode of transmission, especially the aerosol transmission

☆ Contagious nature of the organism

☆ Zoonotic status

☆ Availability of effective preventive measures (*e.g.*, vaccines)

☆ Availability of effective treatment (*e.g.*, antibiotics, passive immunization, post-exposure vaccination, chemotherapeutic agents, *etc.*)

☆ Existing levels of immunity in the population, density and movement of host population

☆ Presence of appropriate disease transmission vectors and standards of environmental hygiene

☆ Risk group categorization and biosafety level classification for pathogenic micro-organisms are provided by various organizations internationally and most of the developed countries had created a system to monitor the compliance of laboratories to the biosafety level requirements.

9.3 WHO classification of infective organisms

Risk Group 1 (no or low individual and community risk)

A micro-organism that is unlikely to cause human or animal disease.

Risk Group 2 (moderate individual and low community risk)

A pathogen that can cause human or animal disease but is unlikely to be a serious hazard to laboratory workers, the community, livestock or the environment. Laboratory exposures may cause serious infection, but effective treatment and preventive measures are available and the risk of spread of infection is limited.

Risk Group 3 (high individual and low community risk)

A pathogen that usually causes serious human or animal disease but does not ordinarily spread from one infected individual to another. Effective treatment and preventive measures are available.

Risk Group 4 (high individual and high community risk)

A pathogen that usually causes serious human or animal disease and that can be readily transmitted from one individual to another, directly or indirectly. Effective treatment and preventive measures are not usually available.

9.4 Biosafety levels

Biosafety levels of the laboratory are determined based on the risk group category of the organism. Criteria for biosafety containment level according to Center for Disease Control and Prevention (CDC), U.S.A.

☆ **Biosafety Level I:** Suitable for work involving well-characterized agents, which are not known to consistently cause disease in immune-competent adult humans, and present minimal potential hazard to laboratory personnel and the environment. *e.g.*: *Lactobacillus spp.*

☆ **Biosafety Level II:** Suitable for work involving agents that pose moderate hazards to personnel and the environment. *e.g.*: Peste des petits ruminants virus

☆ **Biosafety Level III:** Applicable to clinical, diagnostic, teaching, research, or production facilities where work is performed with indigenous or exotic agents that may cause serious or potentially lethal disease through the inhalation route of exposure. *e.g.*: Foot and mouth disease virus.

☆ **Biosafety Level IV:** Required for work with dangerous and exotic agents that pose a high individual risk of aerosol-transmitted laboratory infections and life-threatening disease that is frequently fatal for which there are no vaccines or treatments, or a related agent with unknown risk of transmission. *e.g.*: H5N1 Influenza virus.

☆ The risk perception of the organisms decides the containment requirements and the containment facility will have few or all of the following features, dependent on the Biosafety level classification. This is to prevent the escape of pathogens from the facility which might otherwise result in threat of exposure to the adjacent community and/or personnel handling the organism.

(a) The ability to sustain constant negative pressure to prevent microorganisms from being accidentally released into the environment

(b) Dressing and shower rooms, sealed service areas, specialized doors, entry and exit avenues to prevent cross-contamination, specialized air handling systems with High Efficiency Particulate Air (HEPA) filters, personal protective equipment, biosafety cabinets, *etc.*

(c) Effluent treatment for all the waste materials generated from the facility to render the infectious agents inactive.

(d) Double door autoclaves for decontamination.

(e) The facility would be validated at regular intervals with respect to the compliance of biosafety and bio-security norms

   (f) The laboratory personnel will adhere to strict operational guidelines that are designed to maximize safety and security

   (g) Access to these laboratories is rigorously controlled and monitored

   (h) All the activities of the facilities will be documented and audited periodically.

Containment facility together with strict biocontainment-practices play major role in creating and maintaining biosafety laboratories.

9.5 Biocontainment Facility

The biosafety laboratories should be equipped with primary and secondary barriers for the personnel and environmental protection from the infectious materials.

9.5.1 Primary Barriers

The primary barriers include

   1. Personal protective equipments (PPE) such as gloves, coats, gowns, shoe covers, boots, respirators, face shields, safety glasses and goggles.

   2. Biosafety Cabinets (BSCs)

   3. Centrifuge cups to contain aerosol during centrifugation of hazardous liquids.

If used appropriately, the primary barriers are expected to provide sufficient personnel protection for the handlers from the infectious materials. Most of the operations using the infectious agents are performed inside the BSCs. BSCs use High Efficiency Particulate Air (HEPA) filter to provide various levels of product and personnel protection. Airborne particles and micro-organisms are removed by HEPA filters and most of the containment devices including BSCs, clean room systems and secondary barriers contain these filters. HEPA filter medium is made up of a single, pleated sheet of borosilicate fibers. HEPA filters prevent the passage of most penetrating particle size (MPPS) of 0.3 μm with an efficiency of 99.97 per cent. HEPA filters remove bacteria, spores and viral aerosols from the circulating air. The BSCs are classified as Class I, II and III with increasing levels of environmental protection.

9.5.2 Class I Biosafety Cabinets

Class I BSC uses unfiltered air from the room as the supply air. The exhaust air from the cabinet is filtered through HEPA filters. The exhaust of class I BSC is generally connected directly (hard ducted) to building exhaust and another HEPA filter may be available at the building exhaust side. As the class I BSCs use unfiltered supply air, product protection is not assured (*i.e.* not suitable for sterile operations such as cell culture work). However, environmental protection from the infectious agents is assured with the HEPA filtered exhaust air.

The Class I BSCs are used in animal houses for changing cages, removing bedding materials in cages, grinding infectious tissues, *etc.* They are also used for keeping equipments such as centrifuges and fermentors, which have the potential to generate aerosol.

9.5.3 Class II Biosafety Cabinets

Product as well as personnel protection is achieved using class II BSC cabinets as both the supply and exhaust air is passed through HEPA filters. The functional types within Class II BSCs are A1, A2, B1 and B2. Part of contaminated exhaust air is recirculated depending on the functional BSC type (Table 9.1). The return (recirculated) air is HEPA filtered before recirculation. The HEPA assembly and contaminated air circulation chambers (contaminated plenums) are surrounded by a negative pressure chambers (negative plenum) in type A2, B1 and B2 BSCs. Therefore, the leakages from the contaminated plenums are pulled back into the negative plenum and the escape of contaminated air into the room is prevented. This facility is not available for class I and class II A1 BSCs and leakage of contaminated air into the surrounding room air is possible.

Table 9.1 Class II BSC types

BSC Type	Recirculation	Exhaust	Contaminated Plenum is Surrounded by
A1	70 per cent	30 per cent	Outside air (lab air)
A2	70 per cent	30 per cent	Negative pressure plenum
B1	30 per cent	70 per cent	Negative pressure plenum
B2	0 per cent	100 per cent	Negative pressure plenum

Type A1 and A2 can be connected to facility exhaust through a canopy (thimble connection) which creates 1" gap between the canopy unit and the BSC exhaust filter housing. Exhaust air of the type A2 BSC can also be left to laboratory without connecting it to facility exhaust. In contrast, the type B1 and B2 BSCs are hard ducted to facility exhaust and the air balancing of the facility is performed accordingly. Type B2 BSC exhausts 100 per cent air and there is no recirculation.

9.5.4 Class III Biosafety Cabinets

The completely closed and air tight class III BSC provides the maximum possible containment for the laboratory and environment from the potentially hazardous pathogens. The operations inside the cabinet are performed through glove boxes and the contaminated materials are autoclaved, fumigated or passed through a dunk tank before taking the material outside the cabinet. The supply and exhaust air are passed through HEPA filters and there is no recirculation of air (100 per cent exhaust). The cabinet pressure is maintained negative by balancing the supply and exhaust air volumes accordingly. The exhaust air is passed through a second HEPA filter or inactivation system before releasing it, into the environment. The exhaust is hard ducted for leaving the air outside the building and these ducts are kept away from the ducting systems of the facility. There must be gas tight dampers (closing valves) on the supply and exhaust ducts of the cabinet to permit gas or vapor decontamination of the unit.

Clean Benches (Commonly called as laminar hoods)

Vertical and horizontal laminar flows provide HEPA filtered air over the work space. The unfiltered air from the work surface is released into the room through the front opening of the laminar flow. Clean benches will only provide product protection and does not provide personnel or environmental protection. These vertical and horizontal laminar flows should not be used for handling infectious or hazardous materials (Table 9.2).

Table 9.2: Difference between BSC and Laminar Hoods

Sl.No.	Specification	Biosafety Cabinet	Laminar Hood (Clean benches)
1.	Supply air	HEPA filtered (except for class I BSC)	HEPA filtered
2.	Exhaust air	HEPA filtered	Not filtered
3.	Product protection	Yes (except for class I BSC)	Yes
4.	Environmental protection	Yes	No
5.	Handling pathogenic organisms	Recommended (BSC class II A2, B1, B2 and Class III)	Not suitable for handling pathogenic organisms

9.5.5 Secondary Barriers

The laboratory facility acts as secondary barrier in preventing the escape of infectious materials to the surrounding environment (Table 9.3). The facility should protect the environment and adjacent animal and human community by preventing the accidental release of infectious agents from the laboratory. With higher biosafety levels, stringent biocontainment is achieved.

9.6 Animal Biosafety levels (ABSL)

Biosafety levels are defined for the tests involving inoculation of pathogens in experimental animals (Table 9.4). ABSL I, II, III and IV will provide increasing levels of protection for the personnel and environment against the pathogen.

Apart from the experiments on laboratory animals, activities involving large animals and loose housed animals are covered under BSL-III-Agriculture (or BSL III-Ag). United States Department of Agriculture (USDA) designated high consequence pathogens are also handled in BSL III-Ag. Basic floor plan of the BSLIII laboratory as shown in Figure 9.1.

9.7 Biocontainment Practices

Strict adherence to standard microbiological practices and techniques is a critical requirement for the effective functioning of containment facility. Methods to ensure containment can vary between laboratories due to differences in construction plans and work flow. Therefore, each laboratory should develop a comprehensive biosafety manual that identifies potential hazards and specifies practices and procedures designed to minimize or eliminate exposures to these hazards.

Table 9.3: Infrastructure Requirement for Biosafety Facilities
(Adapted from WHO biosafety manual)

	Bio Safety Level			
	1	2	3	4
Isolation of laboratory	No	No	Desirable	Yes
Room sealable for decontamination	No	No	Yes	Yes
Ventillation				
Inward air flow	No	Desirable	Yes	Yes
Mechanical via building system	No	Desirable	Yes	No
Mechanical, independent	No	Desirable	Yes	Yes
HEPA filtered air exhaust	No	No	Desirable*	Yes
Double- door entry	No	No	Yes	Yes
Airlock	No	No	No	Yes
Airlock with shower	No	No	No	Yes
Anterroom	No	No	Yes	No
Anterroom with shower	No	No	Desirable*	No
Effluent treatment	No	No	Desirable*	Yes
Autoclave				
On site	Yes	Yes	Yes	Yes
In laboratory room	No	No	Desirable	Yes
Double-ended	No	No	Desirable*	Yes
Biological safety cabinents				
Class I	No	Optional	No	No
Class II(A2,B1 or B2)	No	Desirable	Yes	Yes, in conjuction with suit
laboratories				
Class III	No	No	Desirable	Yes, in con junction with cabinent
laboratories				

* Laboratory room is considered as primary containment if the facility is intended for large-scale production of the pathogen (*e.g.* manufacturing units), performing animal experimentation (ABSLIII) and BSL III-Ag. HEPA filtered room air exhaust, anteroom with shower, effluent treatment and double ended autoclave are compulsory in these facilities. If these facilities are not provided, the pathogen can only be handled in primary containment equipments (*e.g.* Biosafety cabinet with HEPA filtered air exhaust) in small volumes

The personnel involved in the handling of infectious agents must be aware of these potential hazards and must be proficient in the practices and techniques required for safe handling of such materials.

Safety practices and techniques must supplement appropriate facility design and engineering features and safety equipment. Following are the suggested

**Table 9.4: ABSL - Summary of Practices and Safety Equipment
(Adapted from WHO biosafety manual)**

Risk Group	Containment Level	Laboratory Practices and Safety Equipment
1	ABSL-I	Limited access, protective clothing and gloves
2	ABSL-II	ABSL-1 practices plus: hazard warning signs. Class I or II BSCs for activities that produce aerosols. Decontamination of waste and cages before washing.
3	ABSL-III	ABSL-2 practices plus: Controlled access. BSCs and special protective clothing for all activities.
4	ABSL-IV	ABSL-3 plus: Strictly limited access. Clothing change before entering. Class III BSCs or positive pressure suits. Shower on exit. Decontamination of all wastes before removal from facility.

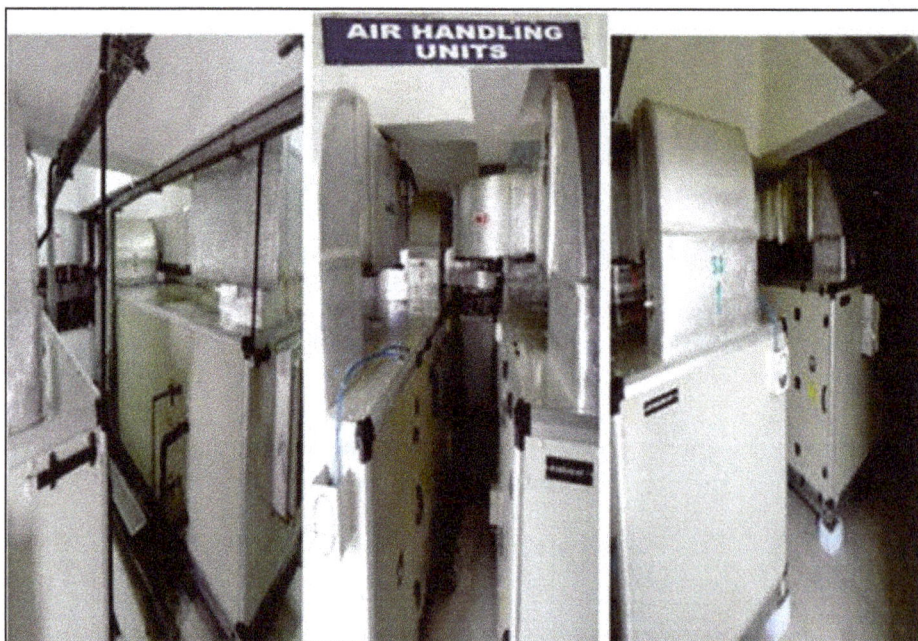

standard microbiological practices to be followed under various biosafety levels. These practices are adapted from the CDC's manual.

Biosafety Level I

BSL I includes following practices:

1. Access to the laboratory must be controlled.
2. Users must wash their hands after working with potentially hazardous materials and before leaving the laboratory. Eating, drinking, smoking, handling contact lenses, applying cosmetics and storing/eating food is not permitted within laboratory areas.

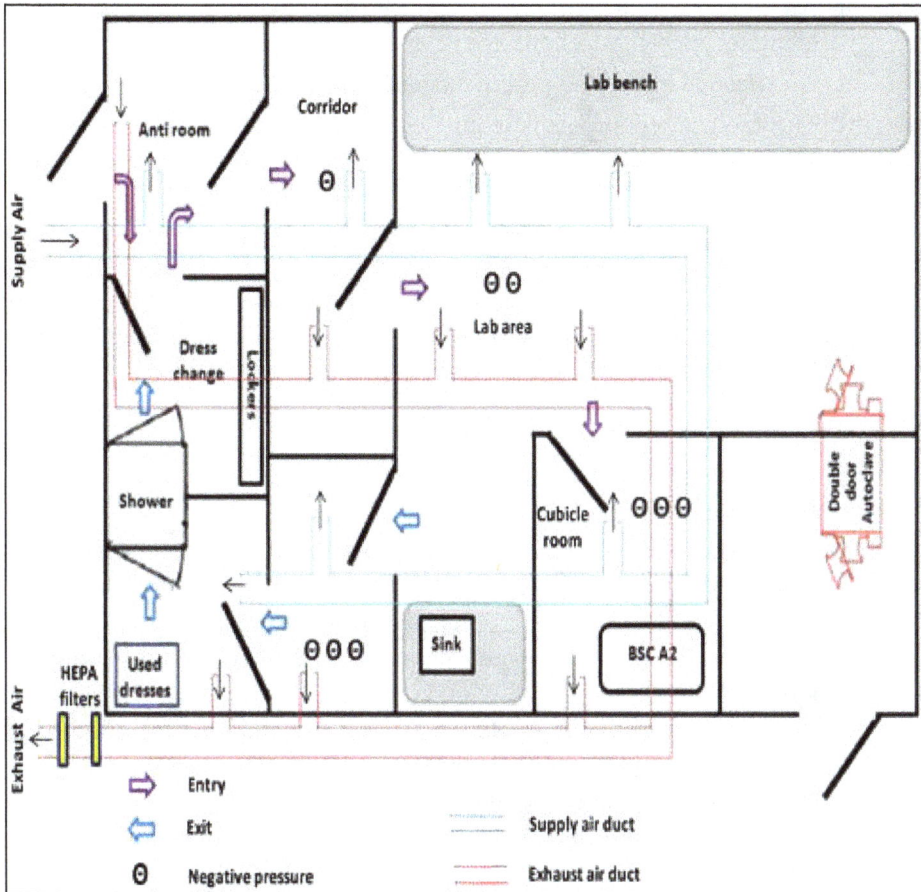

Figure 9.1: Basic Floor Plan of a BSL III Laboratory.

3. Mechanical pipetting devices must be used and mouth pipetting is strictly prohibited.

4. Sharp materials such as needles, scalpels, pipettes, and broken glassware must be safely handled and disposed off in designated waste bins.

5. All laboratory procedures must aim to minimize the creation of splashes and/or aerosols.

6. Work surfaces must be decontaminated after completion of work and after any spill or splash of potentially infectious material with appropriate disinfectant.

7. All laboratory generated materials both biological and non-biological must be decontaminated before disposal using an effective method.

8. An universal biohazard symbol must be displayed at the entrance to the laboratory when infectious agents are present.

9. An effective integrated pest management program should be in place.

10. The laboratory supervisor must ensure that laboratory personnel receive appropriate training regarding necessary precautions to prevent exposures, and exposure evaluation procedures.

11. Protective laboratory coats, gloves are a must to prevent contamination of personal clothing.

12. Protective eyewear must be worn when conducting procedures that have the potential to create splashes. Persons who wear contact lenses in laboratories should also wear eye protection.

Biosafety Level II

BSL II practices include all practices in biosafety level I with addition of the following:

1. All persons entering the laboratory must be informed of the potential hazards and meet specific entry/exit requirements.

2. Laboratory personnel must be provided medical surveillance, as appropriate, and offered available immunizations for agents handled or potentially present in the laboratory.

3. A laboratory-specific biosafety manual must be prepared and adopted as policy. The biosafety manual must be available and accessible.

4. Potentially infectious materials must be placed in a durable, leak proof container during collection, handling, processing, storage, or transport within a facility.

5. Laboratory equipment should be routinely decontaminated. Decontamination is a must after spills/splashes and also before repair, maintenance, or removal from the laboratory.

6. Incidents involving exposure to infectious/hazardous materials must be reported to the laboratory supervisor. Medical evaluation, surveillance, and treatment should be provided and appropriate records maintained.

7. All procedures involving the manipulation of infectious materials that may generate an aerosol should be conducted within a BSC or other physical containment devices. No work with open vessels should be conducted on the bench. When a procedure cannot be performed within a BSC, a combination of personal protective equipment and other containment devices, such as a centrifuge safety cup or sealed rotor must be used.

Biosafety Level III

BSL III practices include all practices in BSL I and BSL II in addition to the following:

1. Entry into the facility must be limited by means of secure, locked doors.

2. While the laboratory is operational, personnel must enter and exit the laboratory through the clothing change and shower rooms except during emergencies. All personal clothing must be removed in the outer clothing change room. All persons entering the laboratory must use laboratory clothing and all persons leaving the laboratory must take a personal body shower.

3. All procedures involving the manipulation of infectious materials must be conducted within a Class II/III BSC.

4. Eye, face and respiratory protection must be used in rooms containing infected animals.

5. Eye and face protection (shield/mask) should be used when performing procedures that can generate splashes or sprays of infectious or other hazardous materials.

Biosafety Level IV

BSL IV practices includes all practices in BSL I and BSL II & BSL III in addition to the following:

1. Entry and exit procedures are similar to BSL III and should be in accordance with the institutional policies

2. Availability of a facility for the isolation and medical care of personnel with potential or known laboratory-acquired infections.

3. The laboratory supervisor should ensure that all laboratory personnel have high level of proficiency in standard and special microbiological practices, and techniques for working with agents requiring BSL-4 containment. All personnel should receive appropriate training in the practices and operations specific to the laboratory facility. Updates and additional training should be done as soon as possible when procedural or policy changes occur.

4. Removal of biological materials that remain in a viable or intact state from the laboratory must be transferred to a non-breakable, sealed primary container and then enclosed in a non-breakable, sealed secondary container. These materials must be transferred through a disinfectant dunk tank, fumigation chamber, or decontamination shower. Once removed, packaged viable material must not be opened outside BSL-4 containment unless inactivated by a validated method.

5. Laboratory equipment must be routinely decontaminated, as well as after spills, splashes, or other potential contamination using an effective and validated method.

6. Only necessary equipment and supplies should be stored inside the BSL-4 laboratory. All equipments and supplies taken inside the laboratory must be decontaminated before removal from the laboratory.

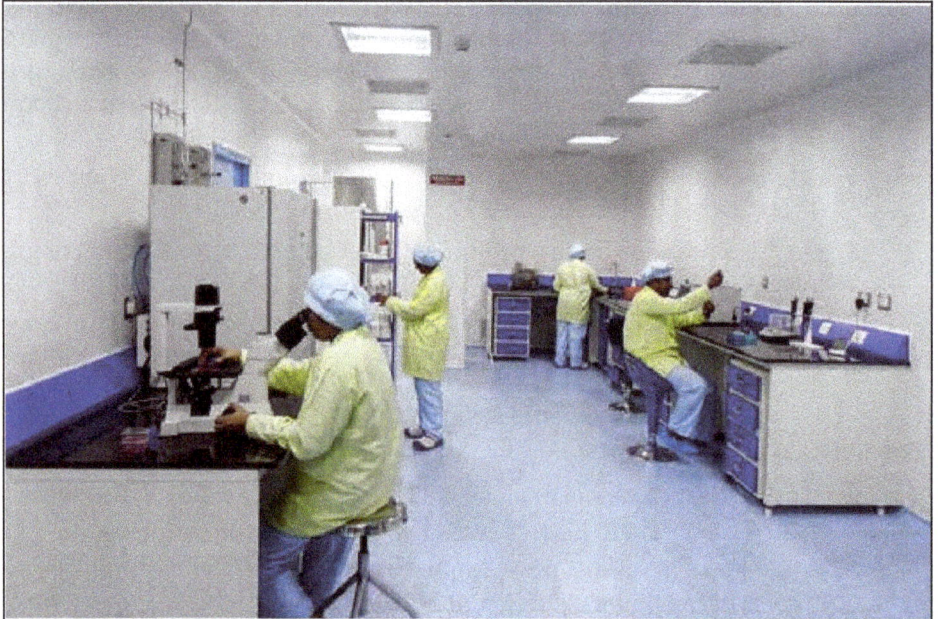

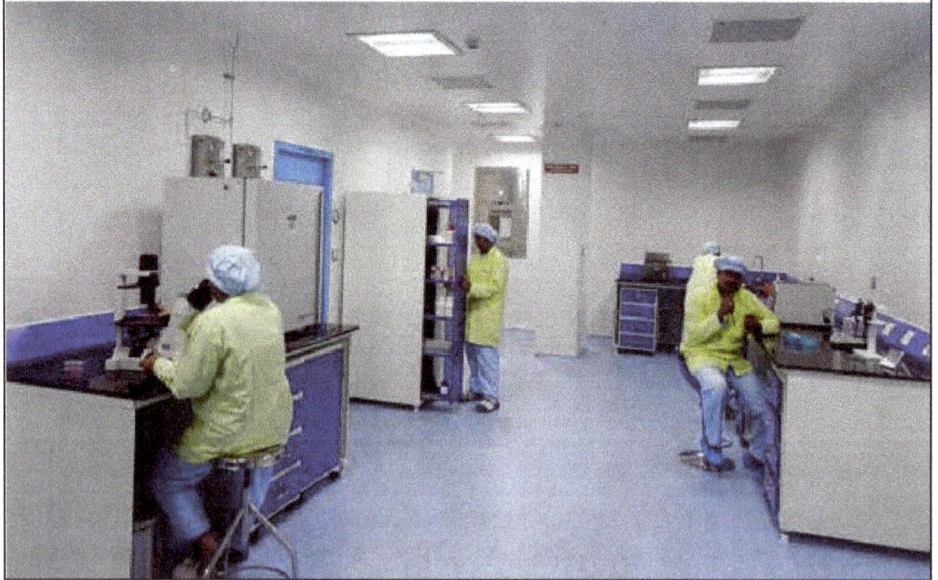

Figure 9.2a: Clean Room Facility Pictures.

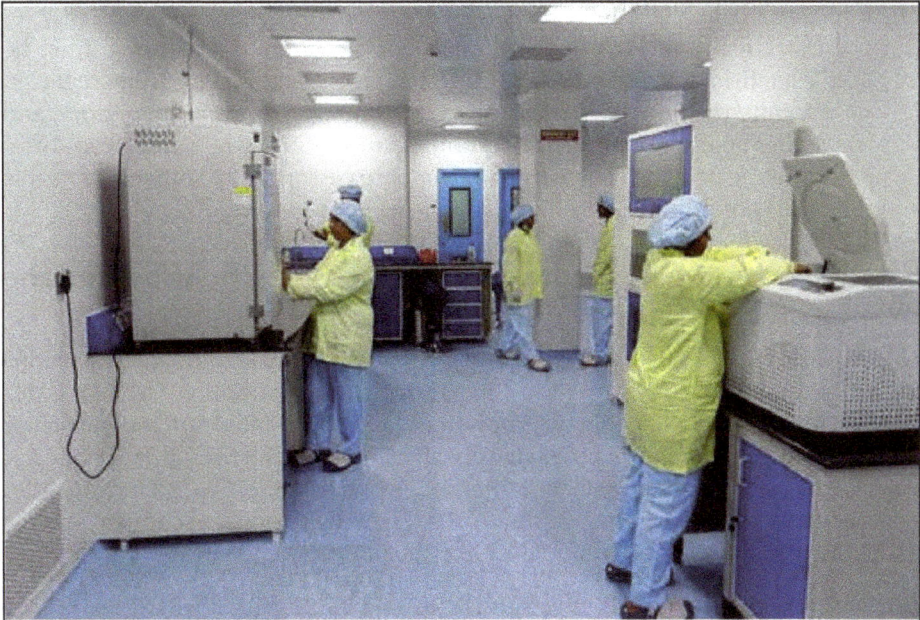

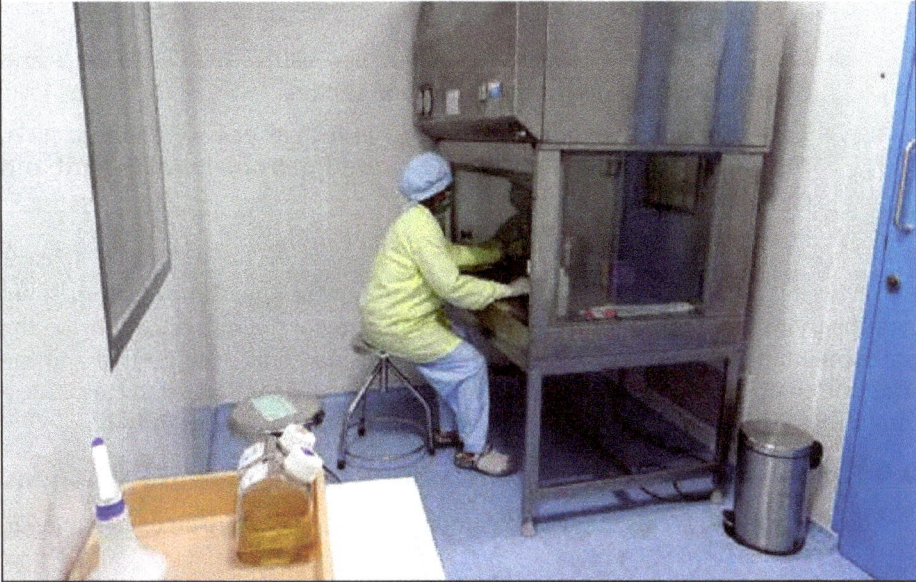

Figure 9.2b: Clean Room Facility Pictures.

7. Daily inspections of essential containment and life support systems must be completed and documented before laboratory work is initiated to ensure that the laboratory is operating according to established parameters.

8. Practical and effective protocols for emergency situations must be established. These protocols must include plans for medical emergencies, facility malfunctions, fires, escape of animals within the laboratory, and other potential emergencies. Training in emergency response procedures must be provided to emergency response personnel and other responsible staff according to institutional policies.

9.8 Requirement of Country Specific Classification for the Biosafety Levels

Biosafety level classifications and practices were developed by various organizations (including American Biological Safety Association (ABSA), CDC, WHO, OIE, *etc.*) and this can appropriately be implemented for the particular country or region. Replicating the same classification and practices in India may not always be feasible. In such instances, alternative practices must be put in place after a detailed assessment of risk. In addition, the following regional or country-specific issues are also to be considered in deciding the biosafety classification.

☆ Existing levels of immunity in the population, density and movement of host population

☆ Presence of appropriate disease transmission vectors and standards of environmental hygiene in the country.

☆ Local availability of effective preventive measures such as vaccines and control of animal reservoirs, arthropod vectors.

☆ Local availability of effective treatments such as passive immunization, post-exposure vaccination, use of antimicrobials, anti-viral and chemotherapeutic agents

☆ Possibility of emergence of drug resistant strains

Therefore, it is important to develop an India specific biosafety level classification. Here, an attempt is made to create such a classification for the common animal pathogens. This can only be considered as a suggestion and the scientific communities in India are welcome to refine these suggestions to create a comprehensive biosafety level classification for animal pathogens in India.

9.9 Biosafety Level Classification for Common Viral Pathogens

Biosafety level classification for common viral pathogens are given in Table 9.5.

Table 9.5: Biosafety Level Classification for Common Viral Pathogens

Pathogen	BSL I	BSL II	BSL III	BSL IV	Remarks
African swine fever virus			-		Exotic agent. Potentially lethal animal disease.
Avian Influenza virus A			-		Serious zoonotic threat. Potential infection by aerosol inhalation. Sporadic in border areas.
Blue tongue virus		-			Prevalent in India with sporadic outbreaks
Border disease virus			-		Exotic and causes congenital and persistent infection.
Bovine immunodeficiency virus			-		Exotic and potentially lethal animal disease causing agent.
Bovine Herpes virus		-			Prevalent in India
Bovine spongiform encephalopathy virus				-	Not reported in India. Potentially lethal disease causing agent.
Bovine viral diarrhea virus			-		Potentially lethal disease causing agent. The virus infection is reported in India.
Canine adenoid virus, adenovirus 2		-			Prevalent in India
Canine Distemper virus		-			Prevalent in India
Canine hepatitis virus	-				Low animal risk agent.
Canine pardon virus		-			Prevalent in India
Cow pox virus		-			Occasional occurrence in India (buffalo pox)
Corona virus enteritis		-			Emerging disease in canine population of India
Classical swine fever virus		-			Prevalent in India
Ebola virus				-	Exotic and potentially lethal human disease agent.
Equine morbidly virus				-	Exotic and dangerous agent. Unknown risk to lab workers. Unknown mode of transmission.
Equine infectious anemia virus			-		Exotic agent transmitted through placenta and body fluids.
Foot and mouth disease virus			-		Aerosol inhalation, rapid spread and economic loss threat
Fowl pox virus		-			Prevalent in India
Herpes virus simian (B virus)				-	Dangerous and exotic agent. High individual and community risk.
Horse pox virus			-		Not reported in India
Infectious laryngestracheitis virus			-		No reports in India between 2005 and present.

Contd...

Table 9.5–*Contd...*

Pathogen	BSL I	BSL II	BSL III	BSL IV	Remarks
Japanese encephalomyelitis virus			-		Potential aerosol transmission. Zoonotic.
Malignant catarrhal fever virus			-		Exotic and highly infectious agent.
Marburg virus				-	Exotic. High individual and community risk
Marek's disease virus		-			Prevalent in India
New castle disease virus		-			Prevalent in India
Nipha virus				-	Exotic and potentially infectious agent. Unknown risk to lab workers. Unknown mode of transmission.
Peste Des Petits Ruminants virus		-			Prevalent in India
Porcine circovirus		-			Reported in India.
Porcine parvovirus			-		Exotic and highly infectious, causing embryonic and foetal mortality in pregnant animals.
Pseudorabies virus (Suid herpes virus)			-		Highly contagious disease causing agent through saliva and nasal secretions. Exotic agent.
Rabies virus*		-	-		High individual and low community risk. Not ordinarily spread. Serious zoonotic threat.
Rabbit haemorrhagic virus/ rabbit calci virus			-		Exotic and low community risk
Sheep and goat pox virus		-			Prevalent in India
Transmissible gastro enteritis virus			-		Exotic agent causing serious illness
Swine vesicular disease virus			-		Exotic agent
Swinepox virus			-		Exotic agent
Vesicular stomatitis virus			-		Exotic agent.

* Diagnostics can be carried out at BSLII with functional type A2 or higher Biosafety cabinet. All the procedures involving the virus should be carried out inside the BSC and centrifuge cups should be used to prevent aerosol generation. Laboratory personnel should have proper immunization records and knowledge of waste disposal mechanism. Production of large quantities and procedures generating aerosols should be carried out at BSLIII.

9.10 Biosafety Level Classification for Common Bacterial Pathogens

Biosafety level classification for common bacterial pathogens are given in Table 9.6.

Table 9.6: Biosafety Level Classification for Common Bacterial Pathogens

Pathogen	BSL I	BSL II	BSL III	BSL IV	Remarks
Actinobacillus spp.		-			Prevalent in India
Bacillus anthraces*		-	-		Zoonotic threat. Transmission through ingestion of contaminated tissues and inhalation of aerosols. Highly lethal disease causing agent.
Brucella spp.#		-	-		Serious zoonotic threat with available treatment. Transmission through air borne droplets, ingestion of contaminated milk, direct contact with infected tissues and fluids.
Bordetella bronchiseptica		-			Prevalent in India
Borrelia burgdorferi				-	Exotic agent with no immunization and proper treatment.
Camphylobacter jejuni		-			
Chlamydia psitacci§		-	-		Highly potential agent causing fatal disease through aerosol transmission
Clostridium botulinum			-		Rare occurrence in India.
Clostridium perfringes type A and C		-			Prevalent in India.
Clostridium tetani			-		Prevalent in India. Potentially lethal human pathogen.
Coxiella burnetti			-		Exotic agent with effective treatment and prophylaxis
Eschericia coli		-			Prevalent in India.
Francisella tularensis			-		Transmission through ingestion and aerosol inhalation
Helicobacter pylori		-			Prevalent in India.
Klebsiella spp.		-			Prevalent in India.
Lactobacillus spp.	-				Non Pathogenic
Leptospira spp.		-			Prevalent in India
Listeria monocytogenes		-			Prevalent in India
Moraxella spp.		-			Prevalent in India
Mycoplasma spp.		-			Prevalent in India
Mycobacterium tuberculosis, Mycobacterium bovis			-		Zoonotic threat and transmission through aerosol; causing fatal disease.
Mycobacterium avium subsp. paratuberculosis			-		Zoonotic threat (Not proven completely) and transmission through aerosol; causing fatal disease.
Nocardia spp.		-			Sporadic occurrence in India.
Pasteurella multocida		-			Prevalent in India.

Contd...

Table 9.6–*Contd...*

Pathogen	BSL I	BSL II	BSL III	BSL IV	Remarks
Pseudomona spseudomallei			-		Exotic agent causing highly communicable disease through aerosol infection.
Rickettsia rickettsii				-	Exotic agent. Aerosol transmission with no immunization
Salmonellaspp		-			Prevalent in India.
Salmonella abortusovis, abortusequi			-		Exotic agent causing abortion
Staphylococcus spp.		-			Prevalent in India; Drug resistant strains (MRSA) in BSL III.
Streptococcus pneumoniae		-			Prevalent in India.
Streptococcus pyogenes		-			Prevalent in India.
Yersiniapseudo tuberculosis			-		Exotic agent. Transmission through aerosols.
Yersinia pestis			-		Exotic agent. Causes serious disease through air borne droplets and ingestion of infected tissues.

* Diagnostics can be carried out at BSL II. Activities involving high production quantities or high concentration of cultures, screening environmental samples from contaminated locations should be carried at BSL III.

\# Routine clinical specimen of animal/human origin can be handled at BSL II. Handling of aborted foetus products and higher concentration of organisms should be performed at BSL III.

§ Sample diagnostics alone can be carried out at BSL II.

9.11 Biosafety Level Classification for Common Parasites

Biosafety level classification for common parasites are given in Table 9.7.

Table 9.7: Biosafety Level Classification for Common Parasites

Pathogen	BSL I	BSL II	BSL III	BSL IV	Remarks
Anaplasma spp.		-			
Ancylostoma spp.		-			
Ascaris suum		-			
Babesia spp.		-			
Cryptosporidium parvum		-			
Dipylidinum caninum		-			
Ehrlicia ruminantium		-			
Echinococcus granulosus		-			
Echinococcus multilocularis		-			
Fimeria spp.		-			
Entamoeba histolytica		-			

Contd...

Table 9.7—*Contd...*

Pathogen	BSL I	BSL II	BSL III	BSL IV	Remarks
Fasciola hepatica		-			Pathogenic to animals upon
Fasciola gigantica		-			environmental exposure.
Geordia lamblia		-			
Leishmania donovani		-			
Taenia saginata		-			
Taenia solium		-			
Theileria spp		-			
Toxocara canis, Toxocara cati		-			
Toxoplasma gondii		-			
Trichinella spiralis		-			
Trichomonas foetus		-			
Trypanosoma *evansi*		-			
Opisthorchis spp		-			
Plasmodium spp		-			

9.12 Biosafety Level Classification for Common Fungal Pathogens

Biosafety level classification for common fungal pathogens are given in Table 9.8

Table 9.8: Biosafety Level Classification for Common Fungal Pathogens

Pathogen	BSL I	BSL II	BSL III	BSL IV	Remarks
Aspergillus spp.		-			Causes pulmonary infections prevalent in India.
Blastomyces dermatitidis*		-	-		Transmission through parenteral mode causing potential pulmonary infections through sporulating mold forms. Rare occurrence in India.
Cryptococcus neoformans		-			Causes meningoencephalitis which is present in India.
Coccidioides spp#		-	-		Potential infection through aerosol inhalation. Rare occurrence in India.

*   BSL II is Recommended for activities with clinical materials, animal tissues, yeast-form cultures and infected animals. Sporulating mold-form cultures already identified as *B. dermatitidis* and soil or other environmental samples known or likely to contain infectious conidia should be handled at BSLIII.

\#   Activities involving handling and processing clinical specimens, identifying isolates, and processing infected tissues can be performed at BSL II. Propagating and manipulation of identified coccidioides sporulating cultures; processing soil or other environmental materials known to contain infectious arthroconidia requires BSL III.

Table 9.9: Biosafety Level Classification for Genetically Modified Organisms

Pathogen	Biosafety Level	Animal Biosafety Level	Laboratory Hazards	Disposal
Adenovirus	BSL II	BSL II (can be moved to ABSL I, after 72 hrs of administration)	Aerosol inhalation	Susceptible to: 0.5 per cent sodium hypochlorite, 2 per cent glutaraldehyde, 5 per cent Phenol or Autoclave for 30 minutes at 121°C under 15 lbs per square inch of steam pressure. Freshly prepared 10 per cent household bleach (0.5 per cent Sodium hypochlorite) is recommended. Alcohol is NOT an effective disinfectant against adenovirus.
Adeno-associated virus (AAV)	Construction-BSLI; Manipulation-BSLII	I (ABSL II, if helper virus is present)	Aerosol inhalation	
Herpes virus	BSL II	BSL II	Aerosol inhalation	Susceptible to: 0.5 per cent sodium hypochlorite, 70 per cent ethanol, glutaraldehyde, formaldehyde, iodine solutions containing ethanol. Freshly prepared 10 per cent household bleach (0.5 per cent Sodium hypochlorite) is recommended.
Lentivirus	BSL II	BSL II (can be moved to ABSL 1, after 72 hrs of administration)	Parenteral inoculation, ingestion, direct contact	Susceptible to: 0.5 per cent sodium hypochlorite, 2 per cent glutaraldehyde, formaldehyde, ethanol. Freshly prepared 10 per cent household bleach (0.5 per cent Sodium hypochlorite) recommended
Poxvirus	BSL II	BSL II	Aerosol exposure via broken skin contact and parenteral ingestion	Autoclave cultures for 30 minutes at 121° C or 250° F (15lbs per square inch of steam pressure)Disinfect with Sodium hypochlorite (1-10 per cent dilution of fresh bleach). 2 per cent glutaraldehye, formaldehyde.
Baculovirus	BSL I	BSL I	Non pathogenic	Autoclave cultures for 30 minutes at 121° C or 250° F (15lbs per square inch of steam pressure). Disinfectants used: Sodium hypochlorite (1-10 per cent dilution of fresh bleach). 70 per cent Ethanol
Escherichia coli (non pathogenic)	BSL I	BSL I	Oral ingestion	Decontaminate all wastes that contain or come in contact with the infectious organism by autoclave, chemical disinfection, gamma irradiation or incineration before disposing.
Saccharomyces Host-Vector Systems	BSL I	BSL I	Skin contact	

9.13 Biosafety Level Classification for Genetically Modified Organisms

Biosafety level classification for genetically modified organisms are given in Table 9.9.

References

Centers for Disease control and prevention, Office of Safety, Health and Environment, Atlanta, USA.

Biosafety manual, World Health Organisation (WHO)

Pathogen safety data sheets and risk assessment, Public health agency of Canada

Risk Group Database, American Biological safety association.

Biosafety in Microbiological and Biomedical Laboratories, 5th Edition. U.S. Department of Health and Human Services, Centers for Disease Control and Prevention. National Institute of Health.

10

Disease Reporting System

10.1 Introduction

There exists a dichotomy in disease reporting in India. Generally reports or incidence of several diseases are published in literature, but the DAHD website indicates that these diseases are not existing/or are not reported in India. This may be due to independent mechanisms of disease reporting that occurs through the Directorate of Animal Husbandry of the individual States and publications that come from State Universities and Research Institutions.

Figure 10.1 depicts earlier system of animal disease reporting in India.

To cover this gap between field situation and Directorates of Animal Husbandry, Government of India (DAHD) introduced a computational program named National Animal Disease Reporting System (NADRS). This system connects each Taluk, Block, District and state headquarters to Central Disease Reporting and Monitoring Unit at the DADF in New Delhi.

The working process of NADRS is shown in Figure 10.2.

10.2 SMS Server

The facility of SMS is also available in NADRS. This server shall be used for sending and receiving alerts in the form of easy and simple messages to the external users. The alerts shall be related to various animal disease outbreaks, methods to tackle and eradicate the diseases, remedial actions, expert advices *etc*. Through the SMS server via mobile service provides various forms of alerts are sent to the stakeholders.

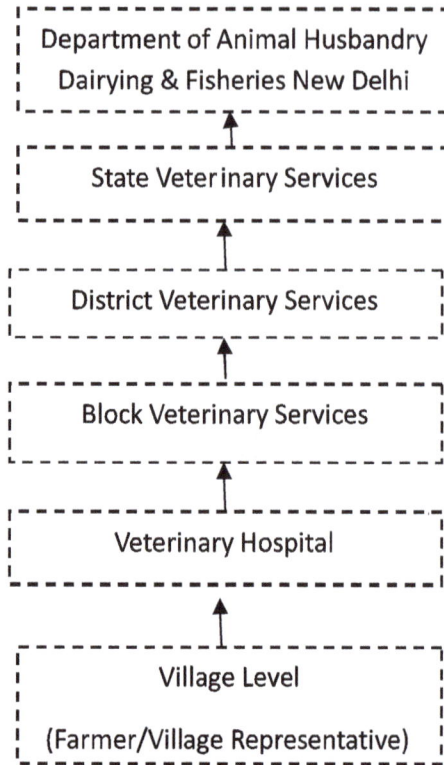

Figure 10.1 Previous System of Animal Disease Reporting.

10.3 Benefits to Livestock Owners

☆ Better management of diseases of their livestock.

☆ Timely availability of veterinary service.

☆ Increased economic gain from higher productivity of animals.

☆ Better market acceptability of their livestock products.

10.4 Benefits to Animal Husbandry Administration

☆ For all stakeholders availability of a common channel for dissemination of animal disease information.

☆ Availability of SMS-based instant alert system for disease outbreaks, spread of diseases, remedial measures and expert advice, enabling prompt control of diseases.

☆ Availability of better decision support system with GIS integration for helpful and timely decision making.

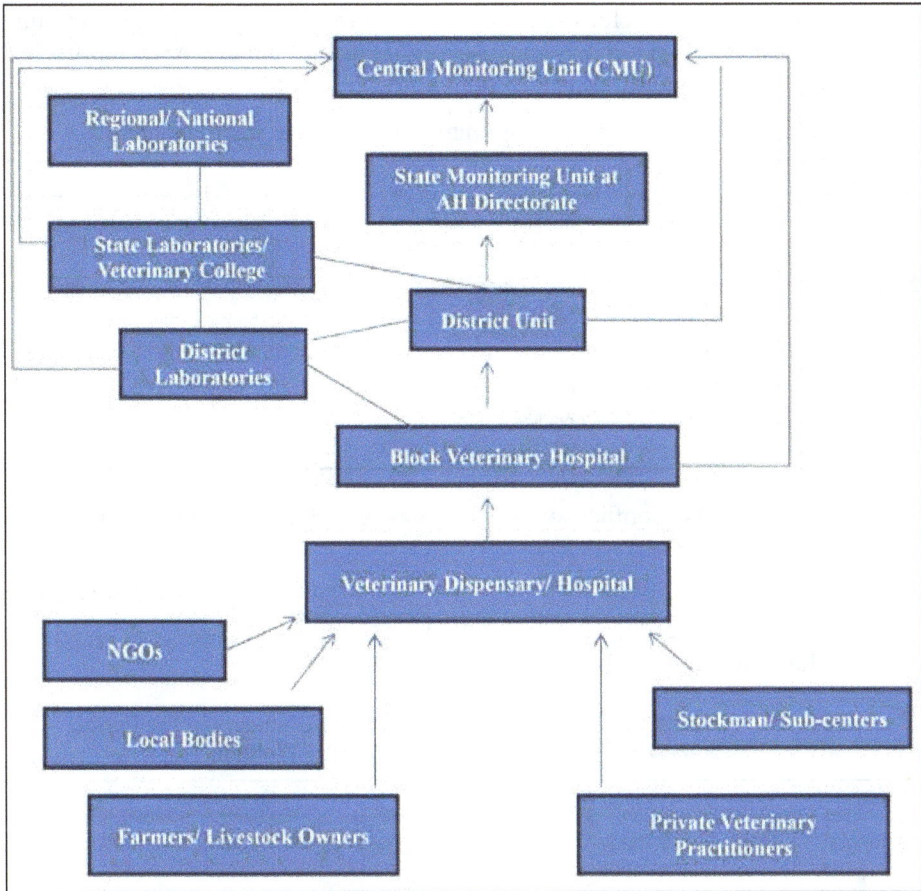

Figure 10.2: National Animal Disease Reporting System Working Process.
(*Source*: Animal Husbandry Department UP website NADRS user manual).

10.5 Benefits to Economy

☆ Improved livestock production and productivity.

☆ Costs of saving otherwise incurred for treatment of animals.

☆ Impulsive growth of the livestock sector, leading to increased employment generation and higher availability of animal protein to the population.

Due to some deficiencies in our old animal disease reporting system some diseases were not reported to Government of India. There are some examples of animal diseases that are reported in literature, but not reported in government website (http://dahd.nic.in/). In these published reports most diseases are detected by presence of antibodies or genome detection which may not be as confirmatory as pathogen isolation.

India has huge market for veterinary vaccines and diagnostics because of huge population of animals in India. Some diseases are not shown in DAHD reports but are having research publications.

Table 10.1: Major Diseases of Animals Reported in DAHD Website

Species	Diseases
Bovine	FMD, Brucellosis, Mastitis, Hemorrhagic Septicemia, Salmonellosis, Babesiosis and Trypanosomiosis
Ovine and Caprine	FMD, PPR, Mastitis, Sheep and Goat Pox, Enterotoxaemia, Babesiosis and Salmonellosis
Canine	Babesiosis
Porcine	CSF, Salmonellosis and Brucellosis
Poultry	Salmonellosis, Coccidiosis, Coryza, Avian Influenza, Infectious Bursal Disease, Marek's disease and Infectious Bronchitis

☆ There exists a conflict between diseases reported in literature and in Govt. DAHD website

☆ An attempt was made to identify diseases that are not reported in DAHD website but available in literature (2009 – 2015)

☆ Reasons for this discrepancy was determined.

Table 10.2: Reports in Literature of certain Bovine Diseases in the Period 2009–2015 not Indicated in the DAHDF Website

Disease	Year	Confirmation Test	State	References
Bluetongue	2015	Antibody detection	Jharkhand	Tigga *et al.* (2015) *Veterinary World* 8.3 346-349.
Bluetongue	2014	Antibody detection	Kerala	Arun *et al.* (2014) *Tropical biomedicine* 31.1 26-30.
Bluetongue	2014	Pathogen isolation	Kerala	Subhadra *et al.* (2014) *The Journal of Infection in Developing Countries* 8.10: 1307-1312.
Bluetongue	2013	Antibody detection	Assam	Joardar *et al.* (2013) *Veterinary World* 6.4: 196-199.
Bluetongue	2013	Antibody detection	Maharashtra	Raut *et al.* (2013) *Veterinary World* 6.7: 416-418.
Bluetongue	2013	Antibody detection	Madhya Pradesh	Sikrodia *et al.* (2013) *Environment and Ecology* 31.2B: 908-910.
Bluetongue	2013	Antibody detection	Madhya Pradesh	Sikrodiac *et al.* (2013) *Environment and Ecology* 31.2A: 694-696.
Bluetongue	2013	Genome detection	Telangana	Rao *et al.* (2013) *Transboundary and Emerging diseases* : doi: 10.1111/tbed.12199.
Bluetongue	2011	Antibody detection	West Bengal	Panda *et al.* (2011) *Animal Science Reporter* 5.3: 105-110.
Bluetongue	2010	Antigen detection	Uttarakhand	Gandhale *et al.* (2010) *Virologica Sinica* 25.6: 390-400.

Contd...

Table 10.2–*Contd...*

Disease	Year	Confirmation Test	State	References
Bovine Papillomatosis	2013	Genome detection	Uttar Pradesh	Kumar *et al.* (2013) *Animal Veterinary. Science.* 1 (2): 53–58
Bovine Papillomatosis	2013	Genome detection	Uttar Pradesh	Kumar *et al.* (2013) *Veterinaria Medicina*, 58 (12): 605–608
Bovine Papillomatosis	2012	Genome detection/ Pathogen Isolation	Uttar Pradesh	Pathania *et al.* (2012) *Transboundary and emerging diseases* 59.1: 79-84.
Bovine Papillomatosis	2010	Genome detection	Uttar Pradesh	Singh *et al.* (2010) *Buffalo Bulletin* 29: 133-134
Bovine Papillomatosis	2010	Genome detection	Uttarakhand	Singh and Somvanshi (2010) *Indian Journal of Animal Sciences* 80: 956-960
Bovine tuberculosis	2014	Genome detection	Gujarat	Parmar *et al.* (2014) *Journal of Foodborne and Zoonotic Diseases* 2.3: 36-44.
Bovine tuberculosis	2014	Genome detection	Madhya Pradesh	Bassessar *et al.* (2014) *Indian Journal of Veterinary Pathology* 38.1: 10-13.
Bovine tuberculosis	2010	Pathogen isolation	Himachal Pradesh	Thakur *et al.* (2010) *Veterinary World* 3.9: 409-414.
Bovine tuberculosis	2010	Pathogen isolation	Karnataka	Phaniraja *et al.* (2010) *Veterinary World* 3.4: 161-164.
Hydatidosis	2014	Pathogen isolation	Maharashtra	Ghodake *et al.* (2014) *Journal of Foodborne and Zoonotic Diseases,* 2.4: 68-71.
Hydatidosis	2014	Pathogen isolation	Punjab	Singh *et al.* (*2014*) *Journal of parasitic diseases* 38.1: 36-40.
Hydatidosis	2013	Pathogen isolation	Punjab	Khan *et al.* (2013) *Veterinary World* 6.9: 647-650.
Hydatidosis	2013	Pathogen isolation	Tamil Nadu	Sangaran and John (2013) *Buffalo Bulletin*, 32 (2): 999-1001
Hydatidosis	2013	Antigen detection	Tamil Nadu	Sangaran and John (2013) *Buffalo Bulletin*, 32 (2): 1009-1010
Hydatidosis	2012	Pathogen isolation	Punjab	Singh *et al.* (2012) *Applied Biological Research* 14.2: 223-225.
Hydatidosis	2011	Pathogen isolation	Tamil Nadu	Sangaran, *et al.* (2011) *Tamil Nadu J. Vet. Anim. Sci.* 7.2: 105-106.
Hydatidosis	2010	Antibody detection	Tamil Nadu	Sangaran and John (2010) *Indian Journal of Animal Sciences* 980–981
Hydatidosis	2010	Antibody detection	Tamil Nadu	Jeyathilakan *et al.* (2010) *Veterinarski arhiv* 80.5: 549-559
IBR	2015	Pathogen isolation	Telangana	Surendra *et al.* (2015) *Advances in Animal and Veterinary Sciences* 3(8): 451-460.
IBR	2014	Antibody detection	Odisha	Das *et al.* (2014) *Veterinary World*: 548-552.
IBR	2013	Antibody detection	Tamil Nadu	Sathiyabama and Ganesan (2013) *Indian Journal of Field Veterinarians* 8.3: 73-74.

Contd...

Table 10.2–*Contd...*

Disease	Year	Confirmation Test	State	References
IBR	2012	Antibody detection	Telangana	Trangadia *et al.* (2012) *Journal of Advanced Veterinary Research* 2.1: 38-41.
IBR	2011	Antibody detection	Uttar Pradesh	Nandi *et al.* (2011) *Transboundary and emerging diseases* 58.2: 105-109.
IBR	2010	Antibody detection	Rajasthan	Gupta *et al.* (2010) *Veterinary Practitioner* 11.2: 169-170.
IBR	2010	Antibody detection	Uttar Pradesh	Singh and Yadav (2010) *Haryana Veterinarian* 49: 54-55.
IBR	2009	Genome detection	Gujarat	Lata *et al.* (2009) *Buffalo Bulletin* Vol.28 No.2: 76-84.
Leptospirosis	2015	Antibody detection	Bihar	Pandian *et al.* (2015) *Veterinary World* 8.2: 217-220.
Leptospirosis	2014	Antibody detection	Gujarat	Patel *et al.* (2014) *Veterinary World* 7.11: 999-1003.
Leptospirosis	2014	Antibody detection	Gujarat	Jignesh Kumar (2014) *Ph.D. thesis* Navsari Agricultural University
Leptospirosis	2014	Antibody detection	Gujarat	Patel *et al.* (2014) *National Journal of Integrated Research in Medicine* 5.4: 22-24.
Leptospirosis	2014	Antigen detection	Uttar Pradesh	Deneke *et al.* (2014) *Molecular and cellular probes* 28.4: 141-146.
Leptospirosis	2014	Antibody detection	Odisha/W. Bengal	Behera *et al.* (2014) *Iranian Journal of Veterinary Research* 15.3: 285-289.
Leptospirosis	2014	Antibody detection	Tamil Nadu	Govindan (2014) *Biomedical and Pharmacology Journal* Vol. 7(1):125-128
Leptospirosis	2012	Antibody detection	Uttar Pradesh	Joseph *et al.* (2012) *Journal of veterinary Science* 13.1: 99-101
Leptospirosis	2012	Antibody detection	Uttar Pradesh	Rana *et al.* (2012) *Journal of Veterinary Public Health* 10.2: 91-96.
Leptospirosis	2012	Antibody detection	Uttar Pradesh	Sachan *et al.* (2012) *International Journal for Agro Veterinary and Medical Sciences* 6.6: 361-365.
Leptospirosis	2011	Antibody detection	Gujarat	Balakrishnan *et al.* (2011) *International Journal for Agro Veterinary and Medical Sciences* 5.6: 511-519.
Leptospirosis	2011	Antibody detection	Punjab	Rana *et al.* (2011) *The Indian Journal of Animal Sciences* 81.2: 143-145
Leptospirosis	2011	Antibody detection/ Pathogen isolation	Tamil Nadu	Nataraja *et al.* (2011) *Southeast Asian Journal of Tropical Medicine and Public Health* 42.3: 679.
Leptospirosis	2010	Antibody detection	Different states	Sankar *et al.* (2010) *Research in Veterinary Science* 88.3: 375-378.
Q Fever	2014	Genome detection	Goa	Das *et al.* (2014) *Infection, Genetics and Evolution* 22: 67-71.

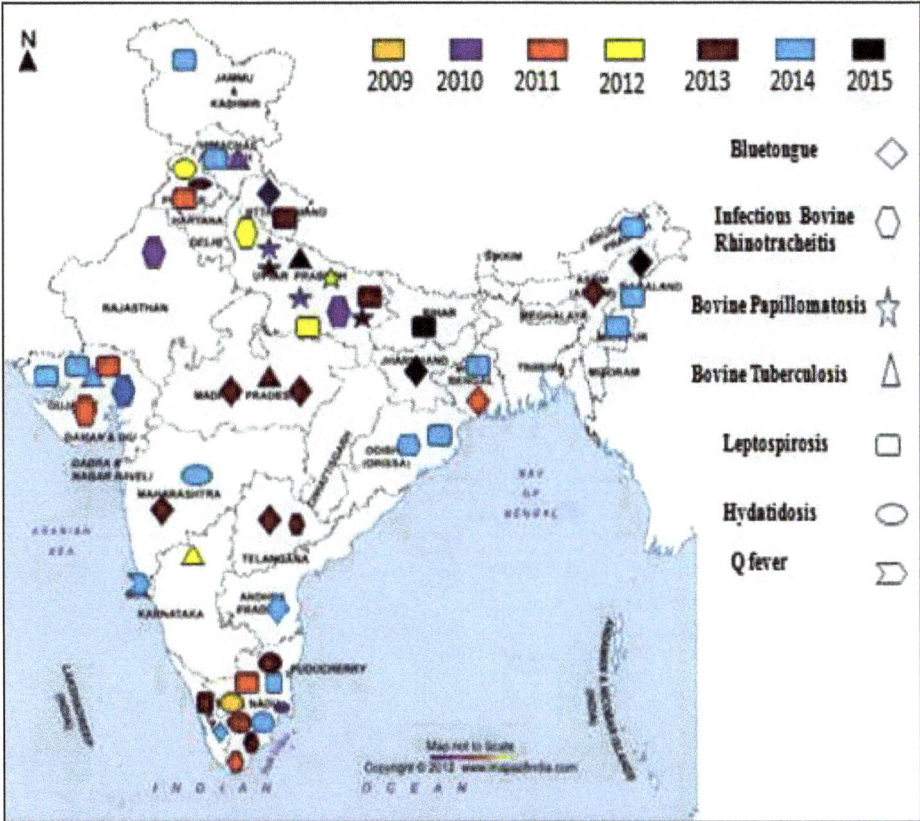

Figure 10.3: Reports of Bovine Diseases (2009–2015) not Reported in DAHDF Website.

Table 10.3: Reports in Literature of Certain Small Ruminant Diseases in the period 2009–2015 not Indicated in the DAHDF Website

Disease	Year	Confirmation Test	State	References
Hydatidosis	2014	Pathogen isolation	Jammu and Kashmir	Godara *et al.* (2014) *Journal of Parasitic diseases* 38. (1): 73-76.
Hydatidosis	2014	Pathogen isolation	Punjab	Singh *et al.* (2014) *Journal of Parasitic Diseases* 38. (1): 36-40.
Hydatidosis	2011	Pathogen isolation	Uttar Pradesh	Gupta *et al.* (2011) *Journal of Veterinary Public Health* 9. (1): 55-57.
Hydatidosis	2009	Pathogen isolation	Tamil Nadu	Sangaranand Lalitha (2009) *Tamil Nadu Journal of Veterinary and Animal Sciences* 5.5: 208-210.
Q fever	2014	Antibody detection	Puducherry	Stephen *et al.* (2014) *The Indian Journal of Medical Research* 140.6: 785.

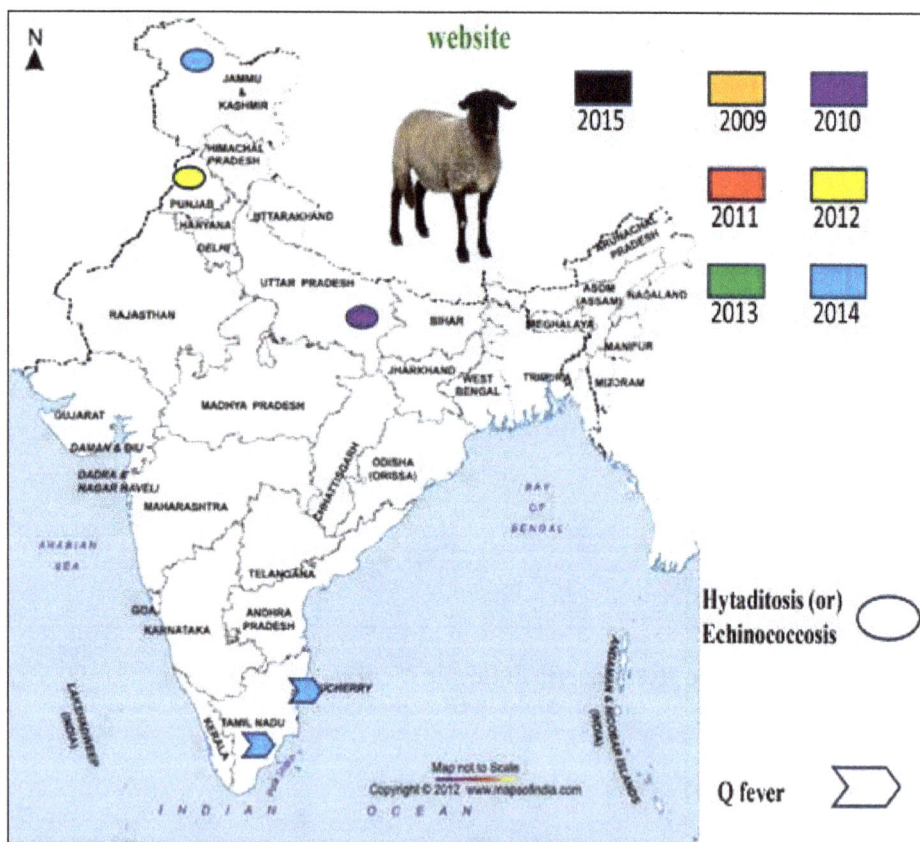

Figure 10.4: Published Reports 2009–2015 of Small Ruminants Diseases not Reported in DAHDF Website.

**Table 10.4: Reports in Literature of Certain Canine Diseases in the
Period 2009–2015 not Indicated in the DAHDF Website**

Disease	Year	Confirmation Test	State	References
CPV	2015	Genome detection	Uttar Pradesh	Singh *et al.* (2015) *The Indian Journal of Animal Sciences* 85.1:12-15
CPV	2015	Antigen/ Genome detection	Kerala	Tinky *et al.* (2015) *Veterinary World* 8.4: 523-526.
CPV	2015	Genome detection	Odisha	Behera *et al.* (2015) *Veterinary World* 8.1: 33-37.
CPV	2015	Genome detection	Punjab	Kaur *et al.* (2015) *Veterinary World* 8.1: 52-56.
CPV	2014	Antibody detection	Maharashtra	Belsare *et al.* (2014) *Transboundary and emerging diseases* 61: 78-86.
CPV	2014	Genome detection	Odisha	Behera *et al.* (2014) *Indian Journal of Veterinary Pathology* 38.4: 226-230.
CPV	2014	Genome detection	Uttar Pradesh	Thomas *et al.* (2014) *Veterinary World* 7.11: 929-932.
CPV	2013	Genome detection	Jammu and Kashmir	Wazir *et al.* (2013) *Veterinary Practitioner* 14.2: 296-297.
CPV	2013	Genome detection	Puducherry	Srinivas *et al.* (2013) *Veterinary World* 6.10: 744-749.
CPV	2012	Antibody detection	Assam	Phukan *et al.* (2012) *Indian Journal of Veterinary Pathology* 36.2: 148-151.
CPV	2010	Genome detection	Haryana	Savi and Prasad. (2010) *Veterinary World* 3.3: 105-106.
CPV	2010	Genome detection	Uttar Pradesh	Kumar and Nandi. (2010) *Transboundary and emerging diseases* 57.6: 458-463.
Leptospirosis	2014	Antibody detection	Kerala	Ambily *et al.* (2014) *International Journal of Advanced Research* 2.7: 684-687.
Leptospirosis	2014	Antibody detection	Kerala	Soman *et al.* (2014) *Veterinary World* 7.10: 759-764.
Leptospirosis	2013	Antibody detection	Kerala	Ambily, *et al.* (2013) *Veterinary World* 6.1: 42-44.
Leptospirosis	2013	Antibody detection	West Bengal	Biplab *et al.* (2013) *Indian Journal of Animal Health*, 52, 1, pp 2730
Leptospirosis	2012	Antibody/ Genome detection	Tamil Nadu	Lakshmipriya *et al.* (2012) *The Indian Journal of Animal Sciences*, 82(7): 702-705.
Leptospirosis	2012	Antibody detection	Uttar Pradesh	Sachan *et al.* (2012) *International* Journal for Agro Veterinary and *Medical Sciences* 6.6: 361-365.
Leptospirosis	2011	Antibody detection	Tamil Nadu	Subathra *et al.* (2011) *Comparative* immunology, *microbiology and infectious diseases* 34.1: 17-22.
Leptospirosis	2010	Antibody detection	Tamil Nadu	Balakrishnan *et al.* (2010) *Indian Veterinary Journal,* September, 87 : 921

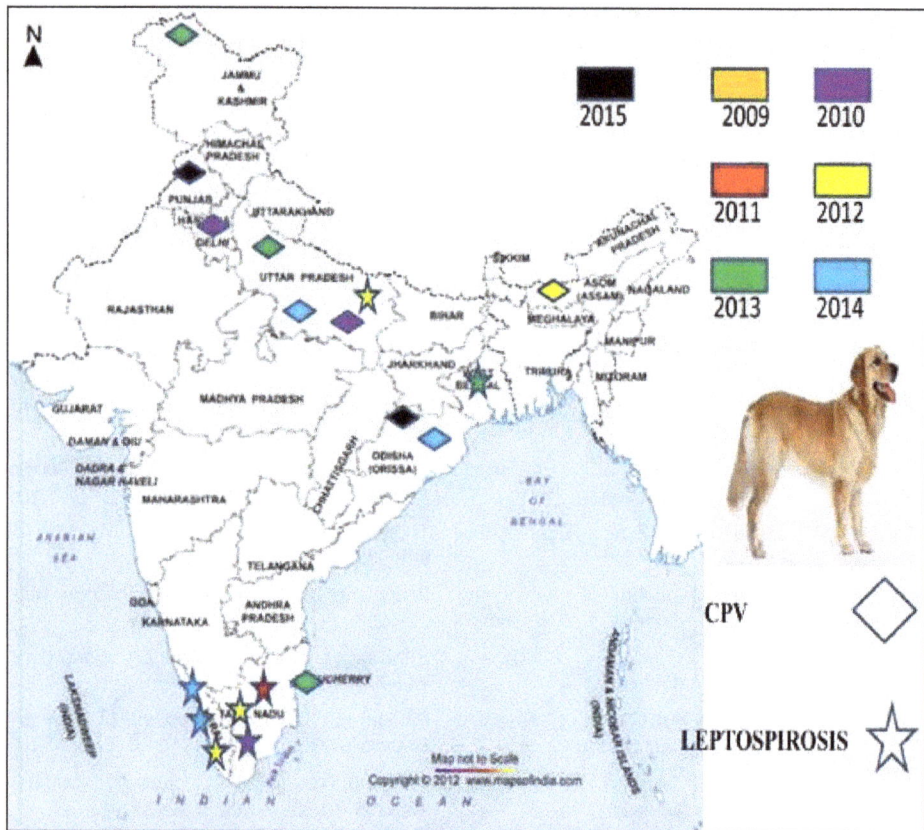

Figure 10.5: Published Reports 2009–2015 of Canine Diseases not Reported in DAHDF Website.

Table 10.5: Reports in literature of certain porcine diseases in the period 2009 – 2015 not indicated in the DAHDF website

Disease	Year	Confirmation Test	State	References
Haemorrhagic Septicaemia	2014	Pathogen isolation	Chhattisgarh	Tigga *et al.* (2015) *Veterinary World* 8.3: 346-349.
Haemorrhagic Septicaemia	2014	Genome detection	Mizoram	Varte *et al.* (2014) *Veterinary World* 7.2: 95-99.
Porcine cysticercosis	2014	Pathogen Isolation	Uttar Pradesh	Saravanan *et al.* (2014) *Veterinary World* 7.5: 281-283.
Porcine cysticercosis	2012	Pathogen isolation	Uttar Pradesh	Rout and Saikumar (2012) *Indian Journal of Veterinary Pathology* 36.1: 94-96.

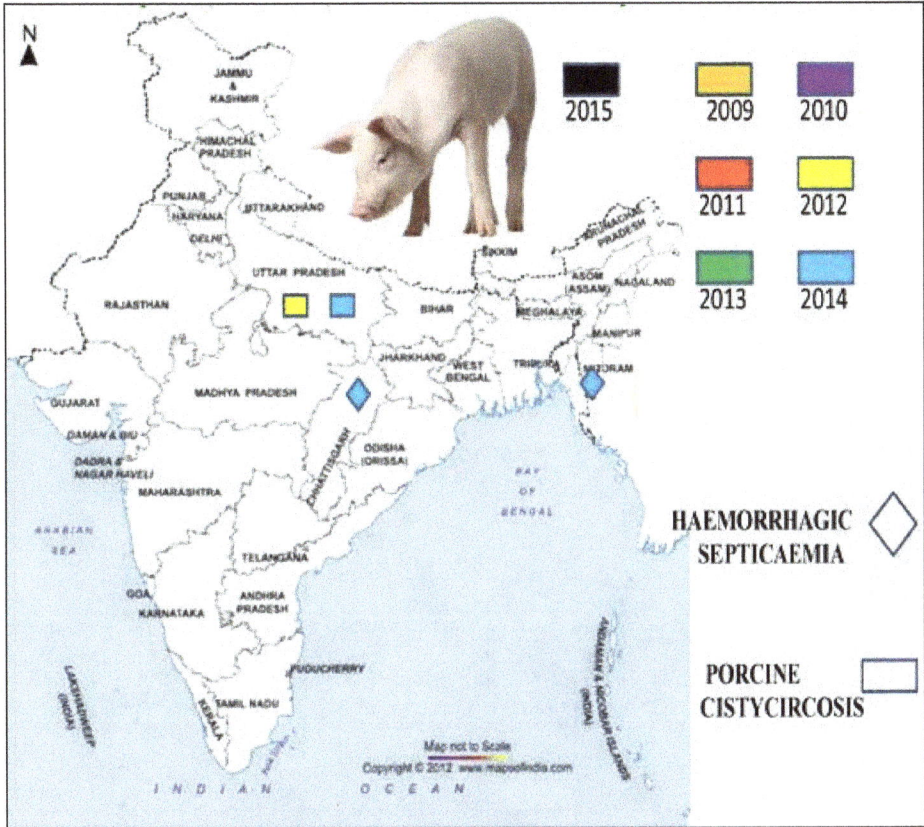

Figure 10.6: Published Reports 2009–2015 of Porcine Diseases not Reported in DAHDF Website.

Table 10.6: Reports in Literature of certain Poultry Diseases in the Period 2009–2015 not Indicated in the DAHDF Website

Disease	Year	Confirmation Test	State	References
Hydropericar-dium syndrome	2015	Pathogen isolation	Odisha	Das *et al.* (2015) *Indian Journal of Veterinary Pathology* 39.1: 46-49.
Hydropericar-dium syndrome	2012	Genome detection	Gujarat	Thakor *et al.* (2012) *Indian Journal of Veterinary Pathology* 36.2: 212-216.
Hydropericar-dium syndrome	2012	Pathogen Isolation	Maharashtra	Sawale *et al.* (2012) *Indian journal of veterinary pathology* 36.2: 255-257.
Infectious bronchitis	2014	Antibody detection	Kerala	Abraham *et al.* (2014) *Journal of Indian Veterinary Association, Kerala (JIVA)* 12.1: 88-90.
Infectious bronchitis	2013	Genome detection	Tamil Nadu	Balasubramaniam *et al.* (2013) *Veterinary World* 6.11: 857-61.
Infectious bronchitis	2012	Pathogen isolation	Tamil Nadu	Balasubramaniam *et al.* (2012) *Indian Journal of Veterinary Pathology* 36.1: 49-53.
Infectious bronchitis	2011	Genome detection	Uttar Pradesh	Sumi *et al.* (2011) *Indian Journal of Poultry Science* 46.2: 226-230.

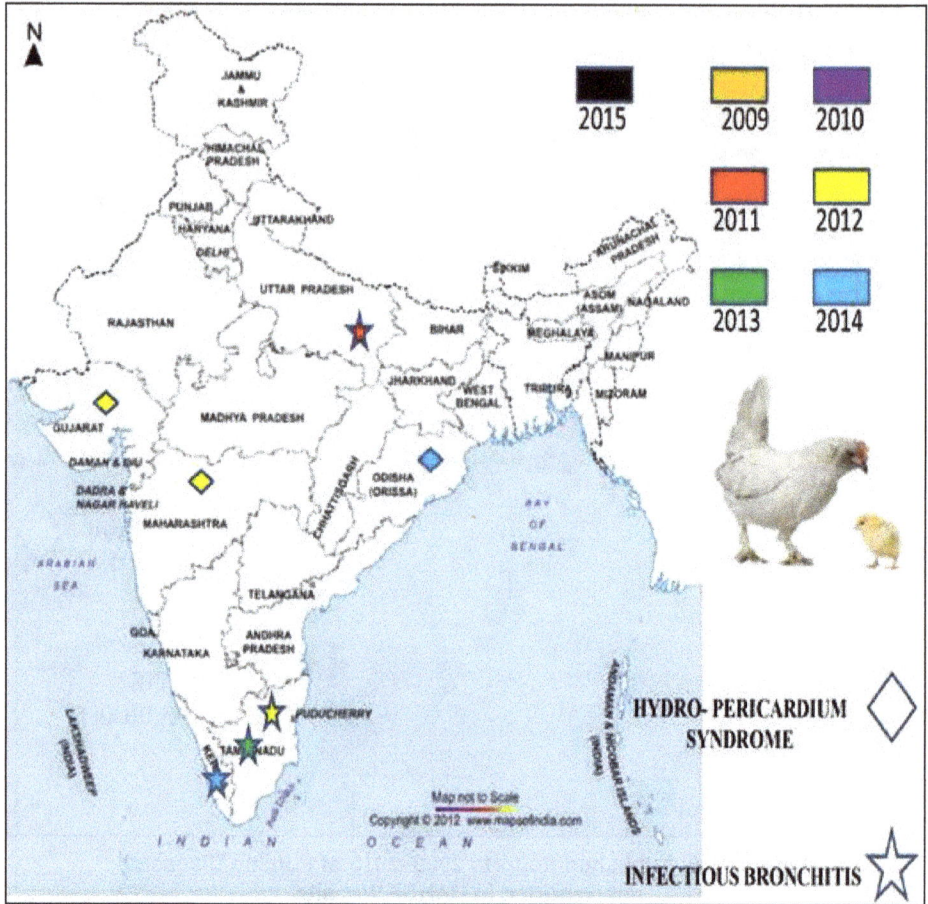

Figure 10.7: Published Reports 2009–2015 of Poultry Diseases not Reported in DAHDF Website.

The mode of confirmation of these individual diseases were compiled as 4 categories and presented in Figure 10.8:

1. Pathogen isolation and identification
2. Antigen detection methods
3. Antibody detection methods
4. Genome detection methods.

Interestingly 45 per cent of the reports were based on antibody detection and only 23 per cent based on pathogen isolation. The pathogens that were isolated before reporting are:

1. Hydatidosis (15 per cent)
2. Hydropericardium syndrome (FAV) (9 per cent)

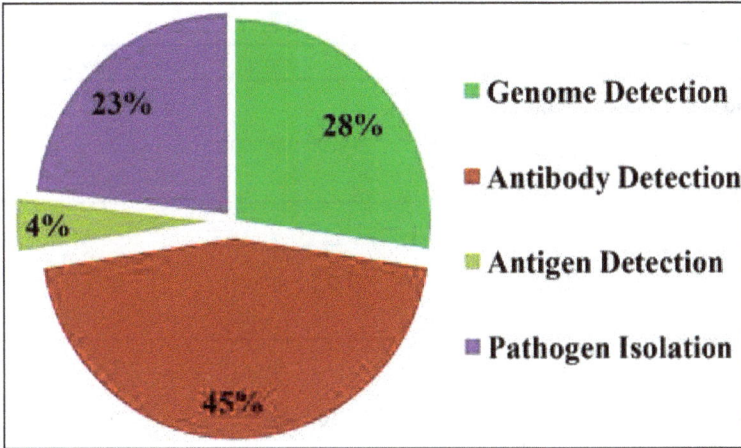

Figure 10.8: Various Methods Used for Confirmation of Animal Diseases (all species) that were Reported in Literature but not Indicated in DAHDF Website.

3. IB (4 per cent)
4. Porcine cysticercosis (9 per cent)
5. HS (4 per cent)
6. TB (9 per cent)
7. Lepto (5 per cent)
8. Bovine papillamatosis (5 per cent) Bluetongue (5 per cent)
9. IBR (5 per cent)

Pathogens reported using other detection methodologies but not isolated are:

1. Leptospirosis(55 per cent) CPV (41 per cent)
2. Q Fever (4 per cent)

Table 10.7: Disease Reports – Journal-wise

Disease	High Impact	Low Impact	No Impact	Total
Bovine diseases				
Bluetongue	2 (20 per cent)	8 (80 per cent)	0	10
Bovine Papillomatosis	3 (60 per cent)	2 (40 per cent)	0	5
Bovine Tuberculosis	0	4 (100 per cent)	0	4
Hydatidosis	3 (33 per cent)	6 (67 per cent)	0	9
IBR	2 (25 per cent)	6 (75 per cent)	0	8
Leptospirosis	5 (36 per cent)	8 (57 per cent)	1 (7 per cent)	14
Q Fever	0	1 (100 per cent)	0	1
TOTAL	**15**	**35**	**1**	**51**

Contd...

Table 10.7–*Contd...*

Disease	High Impact	Low Impact	No Impact	Total
Caprine and Ovine disease reports				
Hydatidosis	0	4 (100 per cent)	0	4
Q Fever	1 (100 per cent)	0	0	1
Canine disease reports				
CPV	3 (25 per cent)	9 (75 per cent)	0	12
Leptospirosis	2	6	0	8
Porcine disease reports				
Haemorrhagic Septicaemia	0	2 (100 per cent)	0	2
Porcine cysticercosis	0	2 (100 per cent)	0	2
Poultry disease reports				
Hydro pericardium syndrome	0	3 (100 per cent)	0	3
Infectious bronchitis	0	4 (100 per cent)	0	4
Total	**21 (24 per cent)**	**65 (75 per cent)**	**1 (1 per cent)**	**87**

☆ *High impact journals are journals listed in Thompson Reuters SCI list, ICAR journals and ICMR journals*

☆ *Low impact Journals are listed in NAAS Rating of Scientific Journals, but not listed in Thomson Reuters SCI (Science Citation Index) list*

No impact journals are Thesis or those not listed in the above list

Interpretation

☆ *Most of the reports are from low impact journals*

☆ *Most of the studies are based on serology*

Disaster Management

11.1 Introduction

WHO defines disaster as any occurrence that causes damage, ecological disruption, loss of human life, deterioration of health and health services on a scale sufficient to warrant an extraordinary response from outside the affected community or area.

Disasters are either natural or manmade. Natural disasters include meteorological, topographical or environmental. Man-made disasters are technological, industrial accidents and security related.

India has striking animal diversity and it is recognized as one among the six main disaster prone nations in the world. The impact and exposure of disaster is high. India is a large country with a humid climate, subject to all type of natural disasters, except volcanic action. 28 per cent of the total cultivable land is subjected to drought and 58 per cent of the total area is prone to earthquakes. Awareness about disaster is essential to protect all animals and mainly important for livestock as the size of the animals dictates the needs to move and shelter them. Livestock owners while constructing their shelter and other buildings should pursue the local building regulations, which vary from region to region depending on the nature of the disaster occurrence area. In the middle of 1996 and 2001, nearly 12 per cent of government income was used on relief, restoration and renovation. Overflows of rivers are the most widespread and disturbing amidst all tragedies that happen in India. National Commission for Floods reports that about 40 million hectares of land is susceptible to flood in India. Usually 18.6 million hectares of acreage is submerged yearly.

Of the total states, about 27 states and union territories are susceptible to disaster. In Andhra Pradesh between November 14 to 20, 1977 cyclone caused unpredictable damage of 2,30,146 cattle and 3,44,056 supplementary livestock. Likewise in Orrisa cyclone in the course of 1982 June, 11,468 cattle were misplaced along with 243 human deaths. Generally, less impact on animals occurs during earth quake, but in the case of Uttarkashi earthquake, 3100 cattle were misplaced beside loss of 770 human lives. About1,02,905 cattle were lost between 1953-1990.

The acting out of the Disaster Management Act, 2005 authorities like National Disaster Management Authority (NDMA), National Executive Committee (NEC) at the nationalized level; State Disaster Management Authority (SDMA), State Executive Committee (SEC) for state level; and District Disaster Management Authority (DDMA) at the district level have been created.

The NDMA created in 2009 under the National Disaster Management Policy, which figure out a variety of economic planning, sectors and system related to disaster aversion, awareness and improvement. Disaster management includes Disaster preparedness, Disaster impact, Disaster response and Rehabilitation and Disaster mitigation.

11.2 Community Based Disaster Management (CBDM)

It is a method which includes sequential phases that can be processed to decrease risk of disaster. Development of CBDM is conducted on the basis of subsidiary, economic scale, integrity, heterogeneity and communal responsibility. CBDM consists of numerous phases like susceptibility risk valuation, planning of reducing risk, prior information system, post disaster assistance, observation and assessment of participants. The CBDM Organizations will be referred with a unique notification or by integrating in the State Acts. CBDM will be called as Village Disaster Management Committee (VDMC) for the rural region and Urban Local Body Disaster Management Committee (ULBDMC) for the urban region (Figure 11.2).

11.3 Impacts of Disasters on Animals

When animals are distressed by disaster, the major problems are food spoilage, zoonotic diseases, animal bites, mental health illness of animal owners due to emotional attachment with animals, high livestock death rate owing to shortage of feed, water and decrease in production.

11.4 Disaster Management Plan for Animals

Considering animals on disaster is very significant as it is essential for the owner who relies on them in developing countries like India. A disaster management plan is necessary for animals which includes:

☆ **Displaying epidemiological study** of the disasters in the area like data collected and interpreted, disaster mapping frequency, total population and risk factor analysis

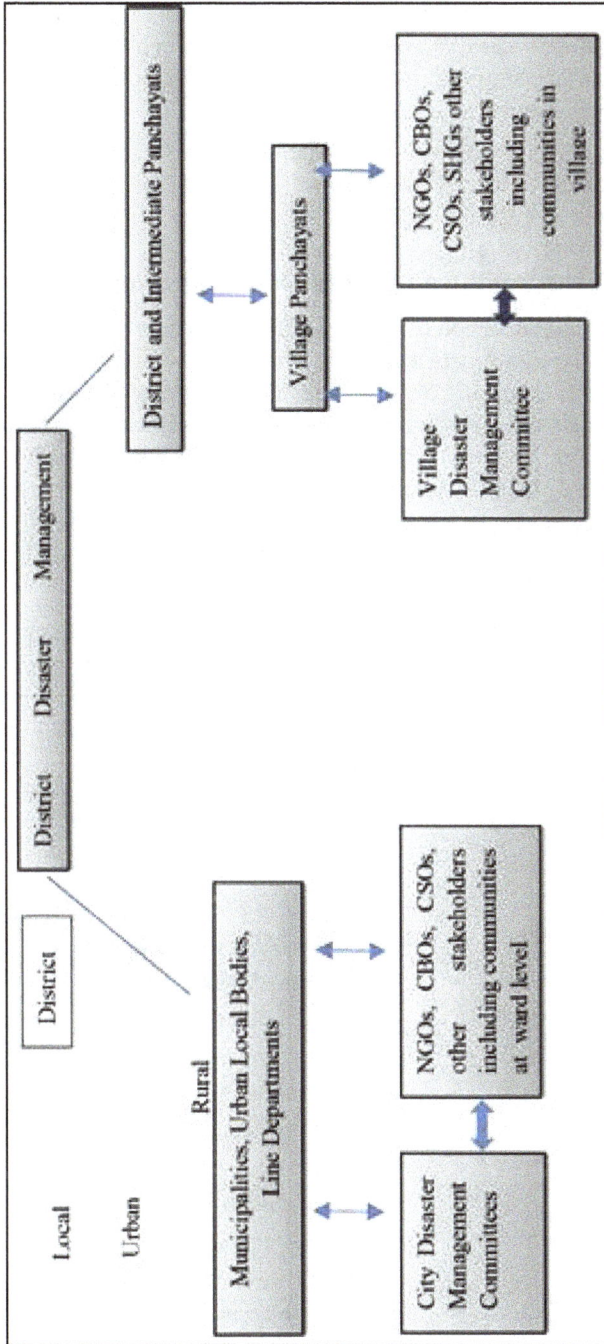

Figure 11.2

Source: National Disaster Management Guidelines, Community Based Disaster Management, February 2014, National Disaster Management Authority, Govt. of India.

☆ **Action Planning on** disaster, animals rescued and collected in relief camps, the immediate priority on controlling and fighting disease. Preventing diseases through vaccination and diagnosing various diseases.

☆ **Planning Resources** like assessing man power such as veterinary doctors, para veterinary staff and includes medicine, surgical appliances and life saving equipments.

☆ **Planning for training** veterinary personnel, administrator and animal health awareness for social workers, volunteers and augmenting political and secretarial support.

11.5 Role of Veterinarians in Disaster Management

During disasters, the function of veterinarians is to secure high values of animal health and to decrease death rate among animals. They can play a main part in promoting pre-disaster planning at district level, which places a high precedence on facilitating livestock and pet migration. Veterinarians have a role to take part in all stages of disaster improvement and management through relief efforts they can play an essential role in increasing the survivability of animals that are wounded, and of those that are used in rescue teams. Their involvement will be most valuable if they combine their proficiency with other limited, nationalized and global groups and firms concerned in disaster management.

Table 11.1: List of Disasters in India during 2012-2015

Month and Year	Place of Occurrence
November 14,2015	Flood in Chennai, Tamil Nadu
October 10,2015	Earthquake in Darjeeling
September 7,2015	Lightening strike in Andhra Pradesh and Orissa
May 13,2015	Earthquake in Nepal
April 22,2015	Heavy storm in Bihar
December 25,2014	Cold wave in North India
September 22,2014	Landslides in Meghalaya
August 11,2014	Flood in Rishikesh
September 23,2013	Flood in Gujarat
September 14,2013	Hail storm in Chennai
August 22,2013	Flood in Odisha
August 5, 2013	Flood in Maharashtra
July 18,2013	Flood in Uttar Pradesh and Andhra Pradesh
June 19.2013	Flood in Kedarnath
May 26,2013	Landslide in Kashmir
December 22,2012	Cold wave in Uttar Pradesh
November 4,2012	Flood in Andhra Pradesh
October 31,2012	Cyclonic storm in Tamil Nadu
September 21,2012	Landslides in Sikkim

Experience has shown that during disasters, the prime anxiety of everybody, and the main aim of every relief measure, is to help people. Though animals are also harshly affected, people must take priority. It is necessary to devise appropriate measures to protect animals and find means to shelter and feed them during disasters and their aftermath, through a community effort to the extent possible.

India launched its first National Disaster Management Plan for Animals on March 3rd 2016 by National Institute of Disaster Management (NIDM), World Animal Protection and Policy Perspectives Foundation (PPF) to ensure that animals are included in disaster preparations which save millions of animals and communities which rely on them.

References

Disaster management: the role and preparedness of veterinary services -E. Mendoza Mainegra, M.I. Percedo Abreu, 2012-OIE

Disaster management in India: the case of livestock and poultry A. Sen and M. Chander. Rev. Sci. Tech. Off. Int. Epiz., 2003, 22 (3), 915-930.

12

Wild Animal Diseases

12.1 Introduction

Two types of wild animals are present in world, free ranging and captive wild animals (wild animals in zoo, sanctuary and national parks). There is lack of information related to diseases of free ranging wild animals however, limited information is available about diseases of captive wild animals.

There are many wild animal diseases that can be caused by viruses, bacteria, parasites and fungi. Some wild animal diseases reported in various publications from India include Rabies, CPV, FPV, CDV *etc.*

Table 12.1: Selected List of Indian Wild Animal Disease Reported in Publications

Disease	Reference
Enteric Bacterial Parasites	Beisner, B. A., *et al.*, 2016 "Prevalence of enteric bacterial parasites with respect to anthropogenic factors among commensal rhesus macaques in Dehradun, India". *Primates.*
Hepatitis E Virus	Nair, V.P., *et al.*, 2016 "Endoplasmic Reticulum Stress Induced Synthesis of a Novel Viral Factor Mediates Efficient Replication of Genotype -I Hepatitis E Virus" *PLoS Pathog.* Vol.12(4).
Surra	Rahman, H., *et al.*, 2016 "Flagellar antigen based CI-ELISA for sero-surveillance of surra". *Vet Parasitol.* Vol. 219: 17-23.
Surra	Banerjee, D., *et al.*, 2015 "Identification through DNA barcoding of tabanidae (Diptera)vectors of surra diseases in India" *Acta Trop.* Vol. 150: 52-8.
Babesia	Bhat, S.A., *et al.*, 2015 "Molecular detection of *Babesia bigemina* infection in apparently healthy cattle of central plain zone of Punjab" *J. Parasit Dis.* Vol.39(4): 649-653.

Contd...

Table 12.1–*Contd...*

Disease	Reference
White Spot Disease	Chakrabarty, U. *et al.,* 2015 "Identification and characterization of microsatellite DNA markers in order to recognize the WSSV susceptible population of marine giant black tiger shrimp, *Penaeus monodon*" *Vet Res.*Vol.25:46.
CDV	Gilbert, M., *et al.,* 2015 "Canine distemper virus as a threat to wild tigers in Russia and across their range" *Integr Zool.* Vol. 10(4): 329-43.
Elephant Endotheliotropic Herpes viruses	Stanton, J.J., *et al.,* 2014 "Detection of elephant endotheliotropic herpesvirus infection among healthy Asian elephants (*Elephas maximus*) in South India". *Journal of Wildlife Diseases Vol.* 50(2): 279-287
Endoparasites	Vimalraj, P.G., *et al.,* 2014 "Endoparasites in cattle nearby tribal areas of free-ranging protected areas of Tamil Nadu state" *J.Parasit Dis,*Vol. 38(4): 429-31.
Classical swine Fever	Barman, N. N., *et al.,* 2014 "Classical swine fever in wild hog: Report of its prevalence in Northeast India." *Transboundary and emerging diseases.*
Anthrax	Chethan Kumar, H. B., *et al.,* 2013 "Occupational zoonoses in zoo and wildlife veterinarians in India: A review." *Veterinary World, Vol* 6:9.
Elephant endotheliotropic herpes viruses	Zachariah, A., *et al.,* 2013 "Fatal herpes virus hemorrhagic disease in wild and orphan asian elephants in southern India" *J Wild Dis, Vol.* 49(2): 381-93
FMD	Pattnaik, Bramhadev, *et al.,* 2012 "Foot-and-mouth disease: global status and future road map for control and prevention in India." *Agricultural Research*1.Vol.2: 132-147.
Tuberculosis	Verma-Kumar, S. *et al.* 2012 "Serodiagnosis of tuberculosis in Asian elephants (*Elephas maximus*) in Southern India: a latent class analysis". *PLoS One,*Vol. **7:**11
Filariasis	Chandy, A., *et al.,* 2011"A review of neglected tropical diseases: filariasis" *Asian Pac J Trop Med,* Vol, 4(7):581-6
CPV	Nandi, S., and Manoj Kumar."Canine parvovirus: current perspective."*Indian Journal of Virology Vol.* 21(1): 31-44.
Blue tongue	Subramanian, K. S. and V. Purushothaman 2010 "A report on incidence of blue tongue in free ranging spotted deer (Axis axis)." *Zoos' Print* 25.4
Infectious bovine rhinotracheitis	Nandi, S., *et al.,* 2009 "Bovine herpes virus infections in cattle." *Animal Health Research Reviews,*Vol 10(1) : 85-98.
Rabies	Sudarshan, M. K., *et al.,* 2007"Assessing the burden of human rabies in India: results of a national multi-center epidemiological survey." *International Journal of Infectious Diseases. Vol* 11(1): 29-35.
CDV	Ramanathan, A. *et al.,* 2008 "Sero epizootiological survey for selected viral infections in captive Asiatic lions (*Panthera leo persica*) from western India." *Journal of Zoo and Wildlife Medicine* 38(3):400-408
FPV	Ramanathan, A., *et al.,* 2007 "Sero epizootiological survey for selected viral infections in captive Asiatic lions (Panthera leo persica) from western India." *Journal of Zoo and Wildlife Medicine,* Vol. 38(3): 400-408.
Newcastle Disease	Roy, P., *et al.,* 1998 "Velogenic Newcastle disease virus in captive wild birds." *Tropical animal health and production,* Vol. 30(5): 299-303
Salmonellae	Sethi, M. S., *et al.,* 1980 "The occurrence of salmonellae in zoo animals in Uttar Pradesh and Delhi (India)." *International Journal of Zoonoses,*Vol.71: 15-18.

12.2 Institutes Working for Wild Animals

12.2.1 Central Zoo Authority

B-1 Wing, 6th Floor, Pt. Deendayal Antyodaya Bhawan, CGO Complex, New Delhi - 110003, Email : cza@nic.in Phone # 91-011-24367846/47/51/52/Fax # 91-011-24367849.

In India, working of zoos is regulated by an autonomous statutory body called Central Zoo Authority which has been constituted under the Wildlife (Protection) Act. The Authority consists of a Chairman, a ten members and Member Secretary. The main objective of the authority is to complement the national effort in conservation of wildlife. Standards and norms for housing, upkeep, health care and overall management of animals in zoos has been laid down under the Recognition of Zoo Rules, 1992.

"Zoo" means an establishment, whether stationary or mobile, where captive animals are kept for exhibition to the public and it includes a circus and rescue centers but does not include an establishment of a licensed dealer in captive animals.

Although the initial purpose of zoos was entertainment, however over the decades, zoos have got transformed into centres for wildlife conservation and environmental education. There are 189 (As on 01/10/2015) zoos in India.

In the recent times, there has been a mushroom growth of zoos in India. Zoos, if managed properly, serve a useful role in the preservation of wild animals. Central Zoo Authority was created for overseeing the functioning and development of zoos in the country. Only such zoos are to be allowed to operate that are recognized and maintain animals in accordance with the norms and standards prescribed by the Zoo Authority.

Role of Central Zoo Authority in Wildlife Welfare

- ☆ Evaluate and asses the functioning of every zoo in India with reference to prescribed norms and standards.
- ☆ Regulate acquisition of animals by zoos, keeping in view the overall interest of conservation.
- ☆ To upgrade technical skills of zoo personnel on various aspects of zoo management.
- ☆ To encourage research with regard to captive breeding and zoo education programmes.
- ☆ To identify endangered species of wild animals for the purpose of captive breeding and oversee their execution including maintenance of appropriate records.
- ☆ To provide technical and financial assistance to zoos for their development and management on scientific line.

12.2.2 Laboratory for the Conservation of Endangered Species (LaCONES)

CSIR-Centre for Cellular and Molecular Biology

Near Pillar No: 162, PVNR Expressway, Attapur Ring Road, Hyderguda, Hyderabad 500 048, Telephone: +91 40 27160222-31, 27160232-41, Email: director@ccmb.res.in.

Laboratory for the Conservation of Endangered Species (LaCONES) is working for conservation of endangered species which was recognized in 2007 with funding from Dept. of Biotechnology (DBT), Govt. of India, New Delhi, Central Zoo Authority of India (CZA), New Delhi and Council of Scientific and Industrial Research (CSIR), New Delhi and Government of Andhra Pradesh. LaCONES was established in 1998 and the laboratory was itself recognized in 2007. The lab would make an effort to: "To promote excellence in conservation biotechnology and serve for conservation of endangered wildlife in India".

Goals and Vision of Laboratory

☆ Development of universal DNA based marker for identification of wild animals from parts and remains or their derivates.

☆ Rehabilitation of smuggled star tortoises based on molecular marker studies to their native ranges.

☆ Development of non-invasive techniques to assess fertility and pregnancy status in big cats and ungulates

☆ Detection of certain parasitic, bacterial and viral diseases in endangered animals from different zoological parks and wildlife sanctuaries in India using DNA-based methods

☆ Development of species-specific microsatellite markers for lion, tiger and leopard to measure heterozygosity and advice zoo management on possible in-breeding

☆ DNA banking of more than 250 species of mammals, birds and reptiles in India

☆ Cryopreservation of gonads from endangered species and their effective revival for production of functional gametes

12.2.3 National Biodiversity Authority

5th Floor, TICEL Bio Park, CSIR, Road, Taramani, Chennai - 600 113 Tel: +91-44-2254 1805 Fax: +91-44-2254 1073, E-mail: chairman@nba.nic.in

The National Biodiversity Authority (NBA) is a government autonomous body under the Ministry of Environment and Forests, Government of India. Headquarter of the organization is situated in Chennai, Tamil Nadu. It was established in 2003 to implement the provisions under the National Biological Diversity Act, 2002, after India signed Convention on Biological Diversity (CBD) in 1992. The organization is working for Conservation, sustainable use of biological resource and fair equitable sharing of benefits of use.

Role of NBA in Indian Wildlife and Wild Animals

☆ Prevent poaching and illegal trade of wild animals.

☆ Make training available for personnel and mobilize financial resources to strengthen captive breeding projects for endangered species of wild animals.

☆ Conservation of wild animals by making wildlife sanctuaries. Regulation of "THE WILDLIFE (PROTECTION) ACT, 1972"

12.3 Other Institutes/Laboratories Involved in Wildlife Health

Centre for Wildlife Conservation Management and Disease Surveillance

Indian Veterinary Research Institute Izatnagar-243122, Bareilly, Uttar Pradesh. Email:aksharmaivri@rediffmail.com Telephone: +91 5812300587, +91 5812586292, Fax: 0581-2303284

Wildlife Institute of India

Post Box #18, Chandrabani, Dehradun – 248001 Uttarakhand, India

E-mail: wii@wii.gov.in

Telephone: +91 135 2640114 - 15, 2646100

Fax: +91 135 2640117

Department of Wildlife Sciences

Madras Veterinary College

Tamil Nadu Veterinary and Animal Sciences University

Madhavaram Milk Colony, Chennai, Tamil Nadu 600051

Phone: +91-44-25551586/ 87, 25554555/ 56, Fax: +91-44-25551576/ 85

http://www.tanuvas.tn.nic.in

Department of Wildlife Science University of Kota

Near Kabir Circle, MBS Marg, Swami Vivekanand Nagar, Kota - 324 005, Rajasthan, India. Website www.uok.ac.in

Email: info@uok.ac.in

Phone: +91-744-2472960

Centre for Wildlife Studies

403, Seebo Apartments,26-2, Aga Abbas Ali Road, Bengaluru – 560042, India

State Forest Research Institutes

Polipather, Jabalpur,

Madhya Pradesh 482008, Phone: 076126 65540

Kerala Forest Research Institute (KFRI)

Peechi-680 653, Thrissur District, Kerala

Ph.Nos:0487-2690100, 2690110 Fax: 0487-2690111, 2690391

E-mail:kfri@kfri.org; Website: www.kfri.res.in

12.4 Vaccination for Wild Animals

Vaccination of captive animals is very important for health of these animals. Some examples are given below for vaccination of captive animals.

Table 12.2: Vaccination of Wild Animals

Wild Animal	Vaccines given
Canine	CDV, CPV, Rabies
Feline	Feline Parvovirus, CDV, Rabies
Elephants	Tetanus, Rabies
Rhinoceros	Leptospirosis, Tetanus
Bears	CDV, Rabies
Deers	Bluetongue, Tetanus

13

Bull Semen Testing

13.1 Introduction

Artificial Insemination (AI) with frozen semen has been confirmed to be the best means worldwide for genetic improvement through dissemination of superior germplasm. This objective can be achieved only if the frozen semen used in AI programmes conforms to the quality standards. For production and distribution of quality semen, it is most important that the bulls used in AI programme satisfy quality norms, bulls are disease-free and semen is harvested and processed in accordance with the standard protocols. The minimal protocols required for production of quality semen should be highlighted. Failure to observe these guidelines could lead to production of poor quality semen making it unfit for distribution to artificial insemination centres.

13.2 Semen Screening Regulation and Disease Security in Bull Station

Genetic improvement of Indian cattle is being achieved through dissemination of superior germplasm by AI using the frozen semen (FS) from superior bulls. The productivity of Indian cattle has improved by the use of AI programmes. However, quality of the FS should be ensured as it bears larger implications on the success of AI programs. Apart from the sperm quality of FS, quality parameters should guarantee:

☆ The disease free status of the bulls

☆ Semen transmitted pathogenic organism-free status of FS.

As per the standard protocol (MSP) of Department of Animal Husbandry, Dairying and Fisheries, following are the minimum requirements to maintain the health of the bulls and quality of the FS.

13.3 Genetic Testing of Bulls

Genetic testing includes karyotyping and testing for genetically transmitted diseases. It is necessary that all animals be karyotyped to rule out any chromosomal defects. The bulls are also subjected to specific tests for identifying some of the genetically transmitted hereditary diseases (Table 13.1). These tests are done by PCR and/or restriction fragment length polymorphism (RFLP).

Table 13.1: Tests to be Conducted for Genetically Transmitted Diseases

Breed	Tests to be carried out
Indigenous cattle and buffaloes	Factor XI deficiency syndrome, Bovine Leukocyte Adhesion Deficiency (BLAD), Citrullinemia
HF and HF crossbreds	Factor XI deficiency syndrome, Bovine Leukocyte Adhesion Deficiency (BLAD), Citrullinemia, Deficiency of Uridine Monophosphate Synthase (DUMPS)
Jersey and Jersey Crossbreds	Factor XI deficiency syndrome, Bovine Leukocyte Adhesion Deficiency (BLAD), Citrullinemia

13.4 Infectious Disease Testing for Bulls

Bulls are to be tested against Tuberculosis, Johne's disease, Brucellosis, Campylobacteriosis, Infectious bovine rhino-tracheitis (IBR), Bovine viral diarrhoea (BVD) and Trichomoniasis. As per OIE guidelines, the breeding bulls should be free from above mentioned diseases. Though Johne's disease is not a sexually transmitted disease but from the herd health point of view, bulls found positive should be removed and therefore it has been included in the MSP. The bulls in the rearing station and the resident herd should go through periodical testing and vaccinations.

Table 13.2: Decision Guide for Culling of Bulls and Discarding Semen Doses Due to the Positive Results for Specific Diseases

Diseases	Bulls	Semen Doses
FMD	Retain	Last one month's doses to be discarded
Brucellosis	Castrate and remove	FS doses in stock to be discarded since the last negative test
TB	Remove	FS doses in stock to be discarded since the last negative test
JD	Remove	FS doses in stock to be discarded since the last negative test
Campylobac-teriosis	Treat and retain	FS doses in stock to be discarded since the last negative test
Trichomoniasis	Treat and retain	FS doses in stock to be discarded since the last negative test
IBR	Preferably remove	If retained, each batch of semen should be tested for BHV 1 and discard positive batches
BVD	Remove	FS doses in stock to be discarded since the last negative test

The semen station must remove bulls (within 48 hours) which are positive for Brucellosis, TB and JD. Bulls found positive for Campylobacteriosis and Trichomoniasis shall be isolated and treated. Besides, the semen station shall cull those bulls which have completed eight years of productive period or 3 lakh semen doses, whichever is achieved earlier.

Table 13.3: Testing Methods for Various Infectious Diseases

Disease	Test	Sample
Brucellosis	ELISA	Serum
Tuberculosis	DTH-Tuberculin PPD/Interferon Gamma Release Assay (IGRA)	Intra-dermal on the bull; IGRA using unclotted blood
Johne's disease	DTH- Johnin PPD, ELISA, IGRA	Intra-dermal on the bull; ELISA from serum; IGRA using unclotted blood
Trichomoniasis	Agent identification	Preputial washings/semen
Bovine Genital Campylobacteriosis	Agent identification	Preputial washings
FMD	ELISA	Serum
IBR	ELISA; Virus isolation; Real time PCR	ELISA from serum; Virus isolation and Real time PCR from semen.

13.5 Vaccination Schedule

The bulls shall be vaccinated against FMD, HS, BQ, Theileriosis and Anthrax. Crossbred bulls shall be vaccinated against Theileriosis once in their lifetime.

The semen station shall arrange for carrying out ring vaccinations against FMD for all cloven footed animals including swine within a radius of 10 km around the semen station. Vaccinations against HS and BQ shall be carried out in the areas having incidence of these diseases.

Table 13.4: Bull Semen Testing Centres in India

Sl.No.	Name	Communicating Details
1.	**Artificial Breeding Research Centre** National Dairy Research Institute Karnal, Haryana, India	Ph : 0184-2259331, 09896125955 E-mail : ak_chakravarty@yahoo.co.in
2.	**BAIF Semen Freezing Laboratory** Dharouli, Jind, Haryana, India	Phone:01686-268563,Fax:01686-268248 E-mail :baifjind@gmail.com
3.	**BAIF Development Research Foundation** BAIF Bhavan, Dr. Manibhai Desai Nagar Warje, Pune, India	Phone : 91-20-25231661/64700562/64700175 Fax : 91-20-25231662 E-mail : baif@baif.org.in
4.	**Sabarmati Ashram Gaushala** National Dairy Development Board Near Gandhi Ashram, Ashram Road, Old Wadaj, Ahmedabad, Gujarat	Phone:+91-79-27557620, Fax:+91-79-27556088 Email: sagho@sagbidaj.org
5.	**Animal Breeding Center** Post Box No. 01, Salon – 229127 Amethi, UP, India	Phone : 05311-274566 Email: info@abc.salon.org
6.	**Regional Frozen Semen Depot** Animal Quarantine and Certification Service Station; Delhi-Gurgoan Rd, Vill Kapashera, New Delhi 110037	Phone: (011) 5563272

Contd...

Table 13.4–*Contd...*

Sl.No.	Name	Communicating Details
7.	**Central Frozen Semen Production and Training Institute (CFSP and TI)** Hessarghatta, Bangalore - 560088	Phone: (080) 8466227
8.	**Genus Breeding India Pvt. Ltd.** **(ABS India)** 406, Amar Neptune, 4th Floor, Plot# 45A and 46, Baner Road, Baner, Pune – 411045	Phone: (020) 65109252

References

http://www.nddb.org.MinimumStandards

http://dahd.nic.in/dahd/WriteReadData/Guidelines_for_export_2013

14

Animal Quarantine in India

14.1 Introduction

The main aim of quarantine stations is to prevent the entry of threatening diseases into the nation through imported domestic animals and livestock products. India is free from several communicable diseases of livestock which are common in foreign countries. So it is, essential that exotic diseases do not get entry into our country through movement of livestock and livestock product beyond the borders. The responsibility of the Office of International Epizooties (OIE) through its International Zoo Sanitary Code is to closely observe livestock disease spread.

The Animal quarantine focus is to prohibit the entry of any non native livestock disease into India through livestock and livestock products importation according to the provisions of Livestock Importation Act (Act No. IX. of 1898) as amended by the Livestock Importation (Amendment) Act, 2001 (5.7.2001) and the regulations orders and SPS standards of the country issued there under. It also helps in providing a globally approved certification for strengthening export and increases the livestock and livestock products in international trade. It mainly examines and records the animal by-product exporting plants. During the fourth five year plan, four animal quarantine stations were established at Delhi, Chennai, Kolkata and Mumbai and over the 11th five year plan, two additional station at Hyderabad and Bangalore were established

14.2 Animal Quarantine Certification Procedures

It is necessary to attain the proper NOC from animal quarantine station prior to transportation of live chicks, pet dogs, cats and other livestock goods (Figure 14.1).

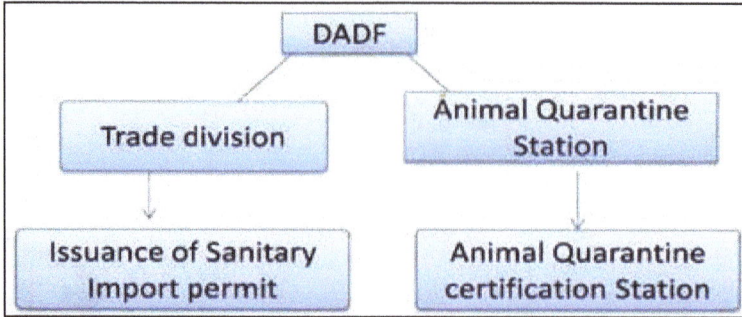

Figure 14.1

Source: Dept of Agriculture and Cooperation, Ministry of Agriculture, 2012.

14.3 Import Issuance of Animal Quarantine Clearance Certificate

The authorized representative should contact the Animal Quarantine Office in advance about the intended import consignment. The same has to be submitted to the office of AQCS in a prescribed format along with photocopies of the Veterinary certificate of animal issued by veterinary officer of exporting country, vaccination details and passport copy of animal owner. Then NOC will be issued by the AQCS office. During arrival at airport/seaport owner should report to the quarantine officer with original certificate. After the custom clearance the quarantine officer will bring the animal to the quarantine station for 30 days for health observation. After completing 30 days, the importer has to contact AQCS office for final clearance.

Livestock products comprise of fresh, frozen and chilled meat and meat products poultry organs and tissues, goat, pig and sheep. It also consists of milk products, egg powder animal origin pet foods and embryos, cow, goat and sheep semen. All these products can reach India with valid sanitary import permit through seaports or airports with quarantine stations.

14.3.1 Laboratories Supporting AQCS

☆ HSADL (High Security Animal Disease Laboratory), Bhopal (imported consignments of Livestock and Livestock products)

☆ NRCE (National Research Centre on Equines), Hisar - (Horses)

☆ CDDL (Central Disease Diagnosis Laboratory) at IVRI (Indian Veterinary Research Institute), Bareilly

☆ RDDLs (Regional Disease Diagnosis Laboratory)

☆ Veterinary colleges

14.4 Export Issuance of Animal Quarantine Certificate

Fitness certificate for export on a required format by the importing country along with filled application will be checked by the quarantine officer.

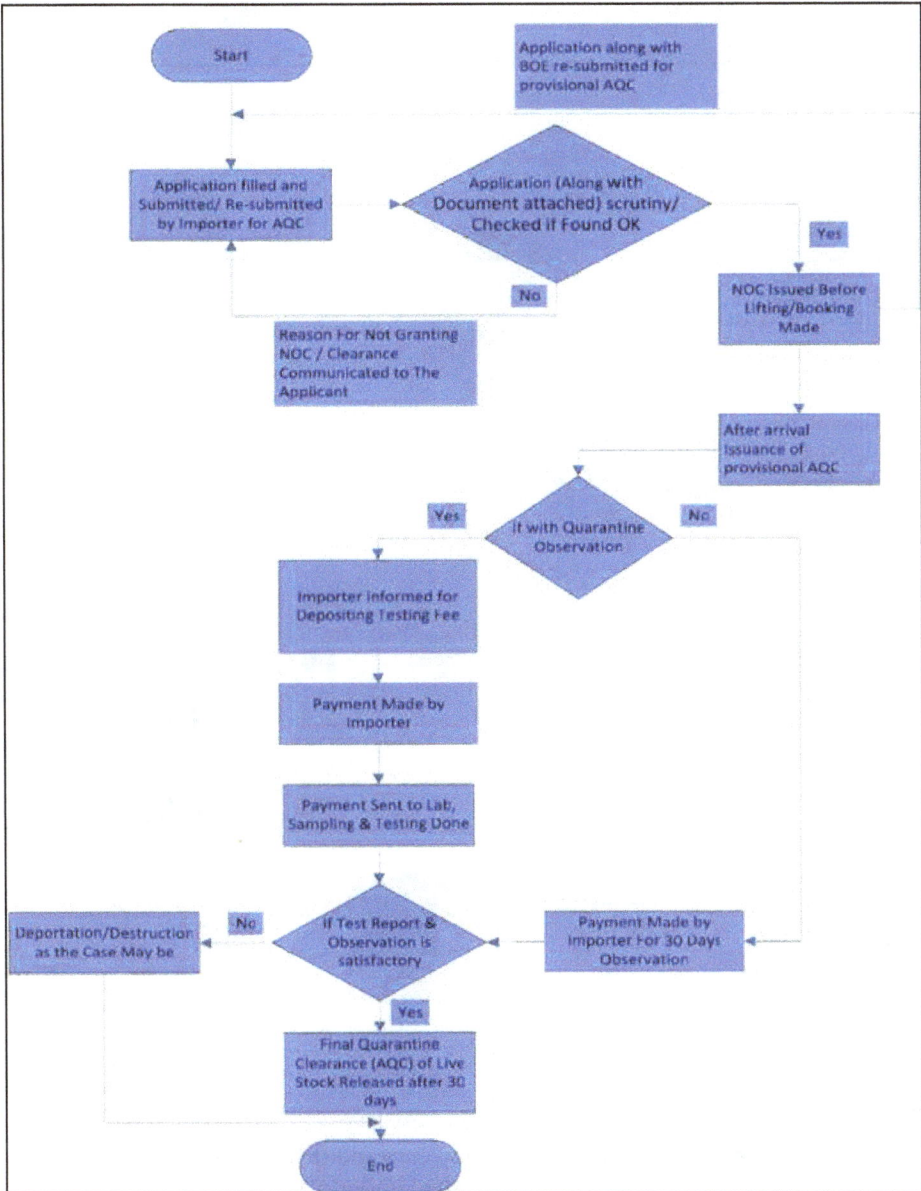

Figure 14.2: Flow Chart of Animal Quarantine Certification for Livestock Import.

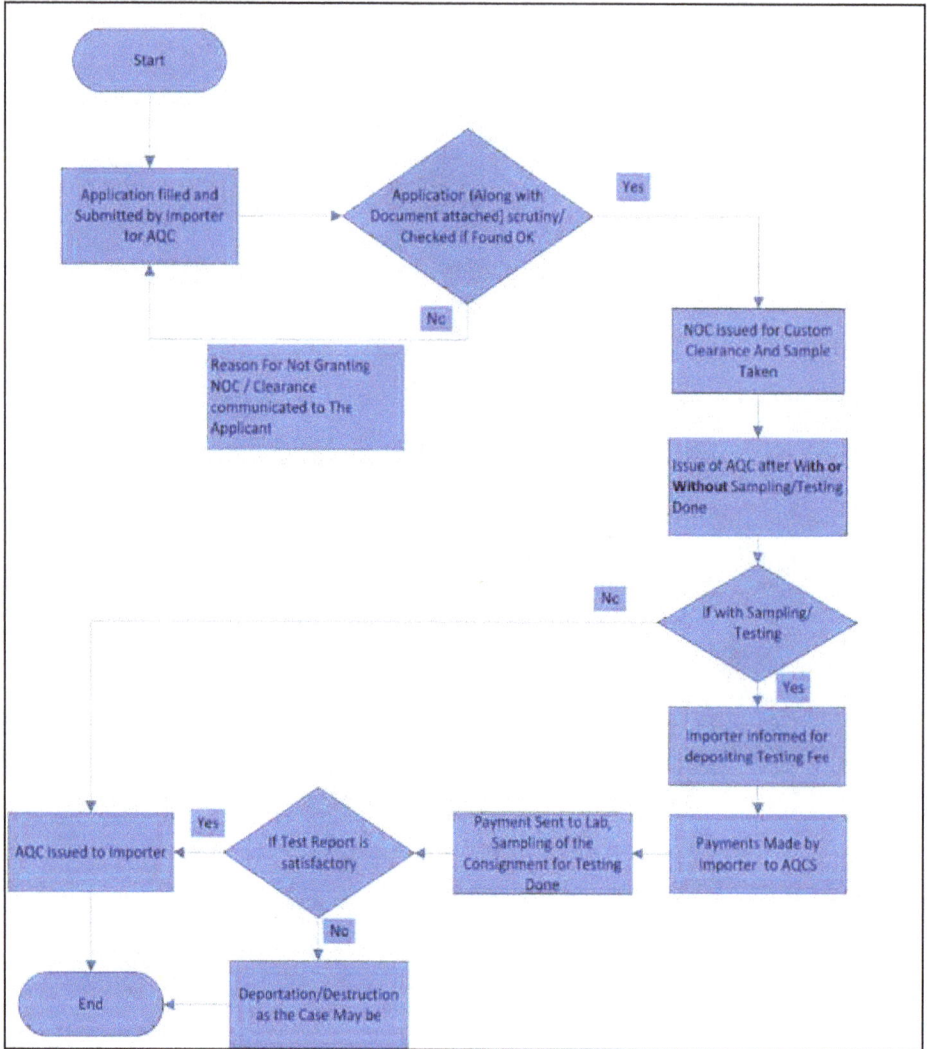

**Figure 14.3: Flow Chart of Animal Quarantine Certification for
Livestock Product Import.**

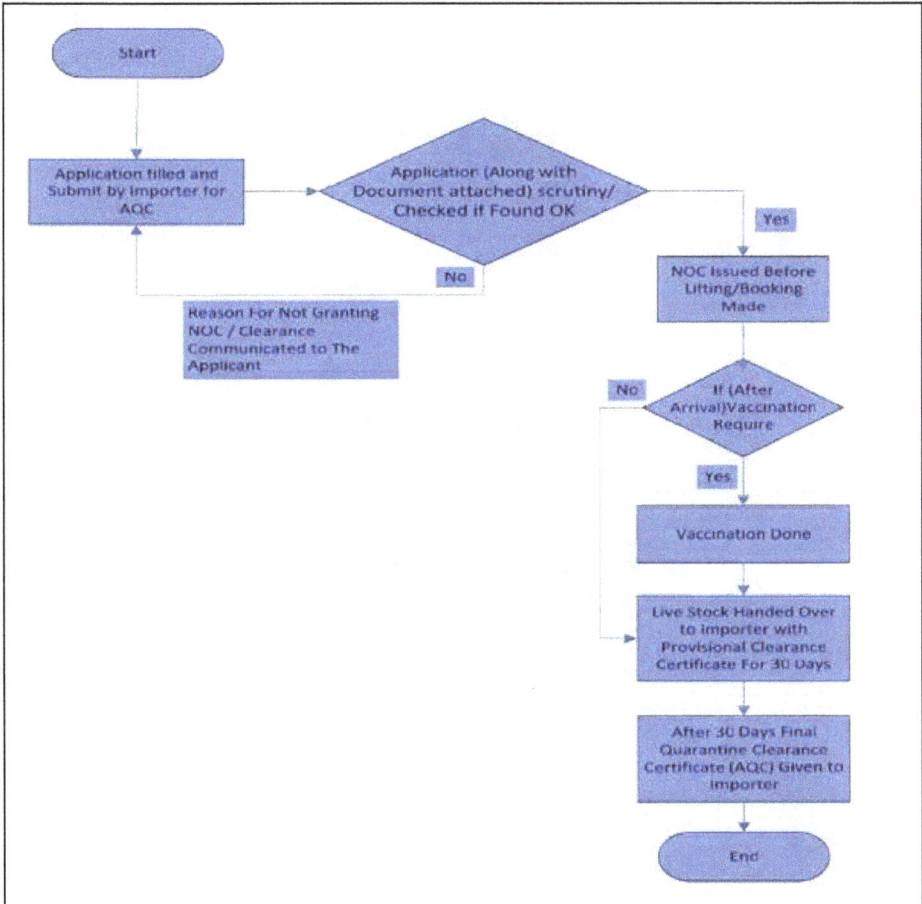

**Figure 14.4: Flow of Animal Quarantine Certification for
Pet Animal (Dog/Cat) Import.**

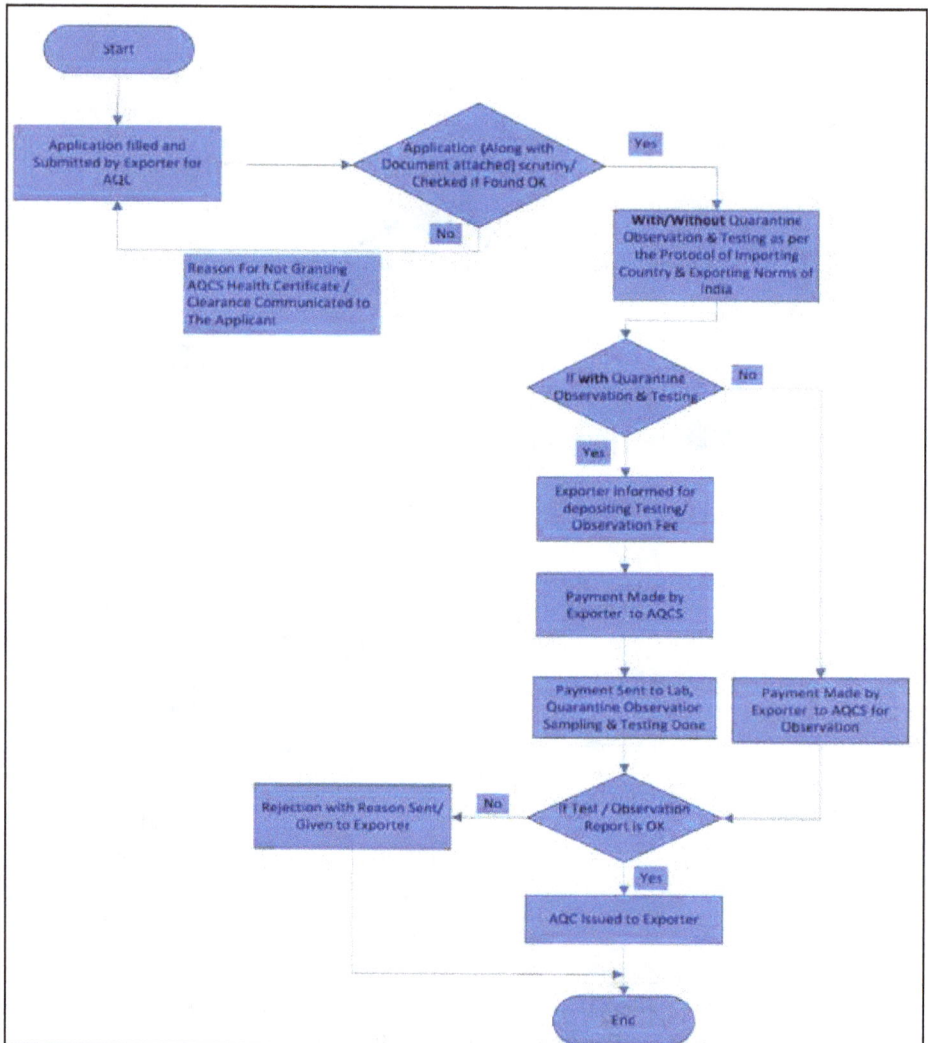

**Figure 14.5: Flow Chart of Animal Quarantine Certification for
Livestock in Case of Export.**

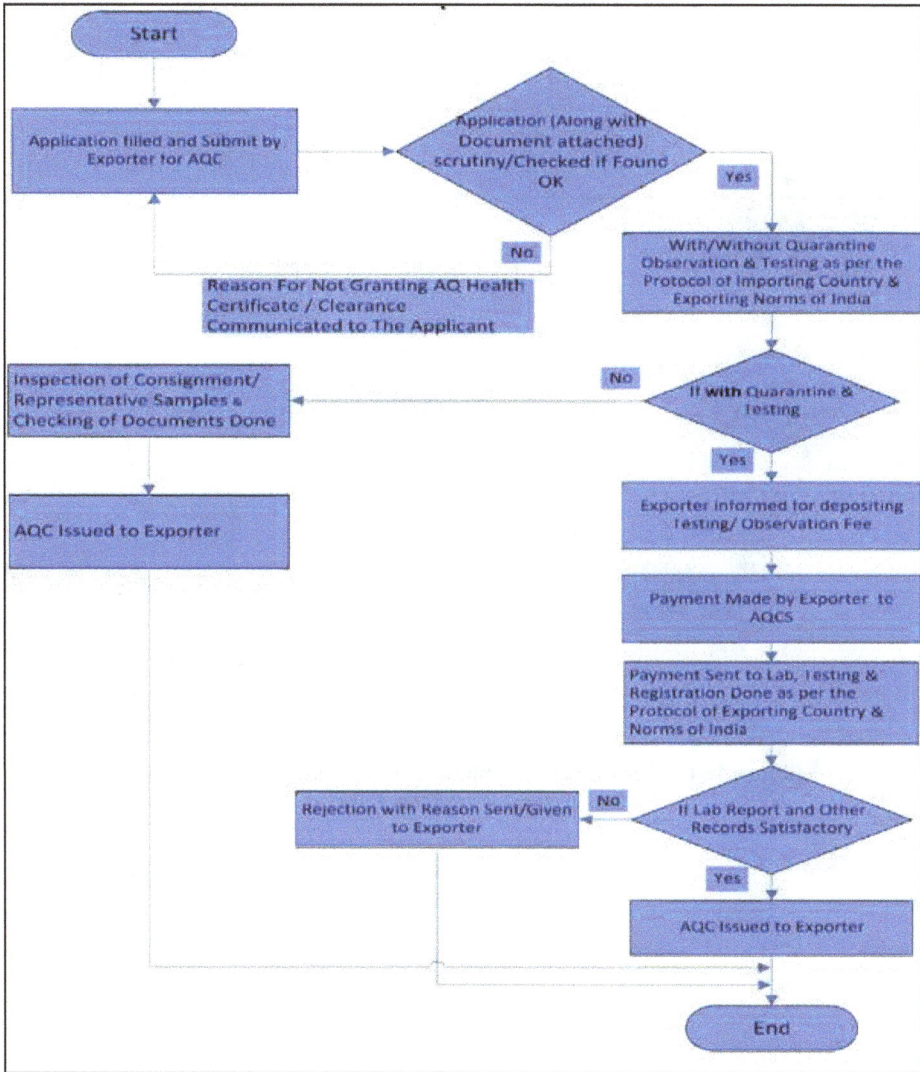

Figure 14.6: Flow Chart of Animal Quarantine Certification for Livestock Product Export.

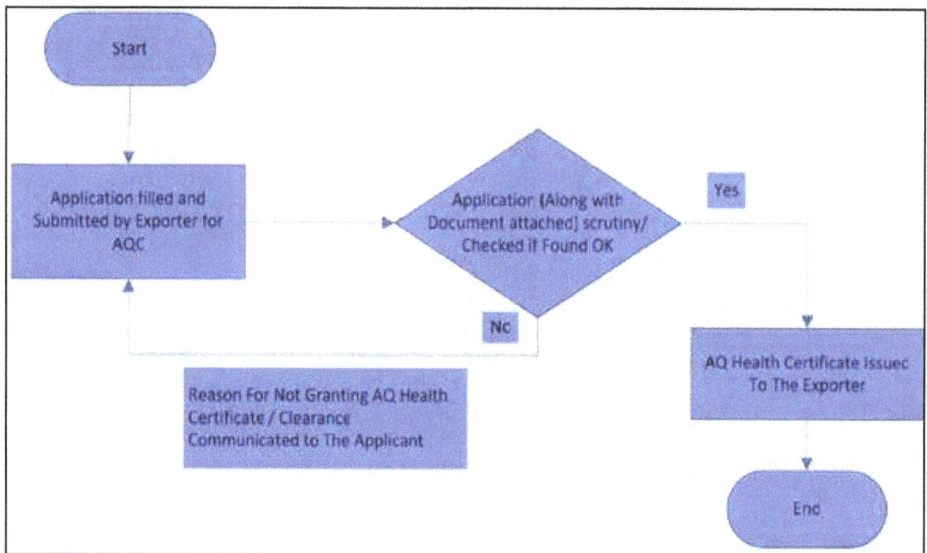

Figure 14.67 Flow Chart of Animal Quarantine Certification for Pet Animal (Dog/Cat) Export.

References

Dept of Agriculture and Cooperation, Ministry of Agriculture, 2012

Animal Quarantine and Certification Services, Govt. of India

Glossary

Antigen: A foreign substance which induce immune response.

Antibody: Immunoglobulin helps removing foreign substances.

Biologicals: Medicinal preparations made from living organisms and their products, including serums, vaccines, antigens, antitoxins, *etc.*

Bluetongue: Bluetongue disease is a non-contagious, insect-borne, viral disease of ruminants, mainly sheep and less frequently cattle, goats, buffalo, deer,dromedaries, and antelope. It is caused by the Bluetongue virus (BTV).

Bovine: The biological subfamily Bovinae includes a diverse group of 10 genera of medium to large-sized ungulates, including domestic cattle, bison, African buffalo, the water buffalo, the yak, and the four-horned and spiral-horned antelopes.

Biosafety: Preventing the harmful organisms from escaping from the laboratory and protecting the handlers and environment from the organisms.

Canine: Anatomy, Zoology. of or relating to the four pointed teeth, especially prominent in dogs, situated one on each side of each jaw, next to the incisors.

CAGR: The compound annual growth rate (CAGR) is the mean annual growth time of an investment over a precise phase of time longer than one year. .

Companion animals: Pet/other domestic animal.

Caprine: Subfamily Caprinae is part of the ruminant family Bovidae, consisting of mostly medium-sized bovids. Its members are commonly referred to as goat-antelopes or caprids.

Canine: Resembling/relating to dog.

Clinical Trail: Research study in which people subject to test new treatments, interventions.

CPV: Canine parvovirus (CPV) is a highly contagious viral disease of dogs that commonly causes acute gastrointestinal illness in puppies.

Crossbreeding: Produce a new one by hybridizing two different varieties .

Diagnostics: Techniques used to help identify a disease, illness, or problem.

Disease: Illness of people/animal.

Disaster: Unexpected accident that causes prominent damage .

Drugs: A medicine introduced in to a body.

Exotic: Introduced from foreign.

Export: Goods to another country for commodity.

Epidemiology: The division of medicine which deals with the occurrence, distribution, and possible control of diseases and other factors describing health.

Feline: Members of cat family.

FMD: Foot-and-Mouth Disease (FMD) is a highly contagious viral vesicular disease of cloven-hoofed animals.

Guidelines: A general rule/principle.

Genome: A total set of genes/genetic in a cell.

HEPA: High-efficiency particulate air, is a kind of air filter.

Import: Goods into a country from abroad for commodity.

Licensing Authority : Permitting to do something.

Mastitis: Mastitis in dairy cattle is the persistent, inflammatory reaction of the udder tissue. Mastitis, a potentially fatal mammary gland infection, is the most common disease in dairy cattle.

New Castle Disease: Newcastle disease is a contagious bird disease affecting many domestic and wild avian species; it is transmissible to humans.

Ovine: Relating to or resembling sheep.

Oligopolistic: Industry/Market influenced by small number of sellers.

Pathogen: Microorganism which can cause disease.

Pharmacopeia: Publication consisting list of medicinal drugs with its effects and direction usage.

Pharmacodynamics: Drug effect and their method of action.

Porcine: Resembling a pig.

Poultry: Poultry are domesticated birds kept by humans for the eggs they produce, their meat, their feathers, or sometimes as pets.

Population: All residents of a particular place.

PPR: Ovine rinderpest, also commonly known as peste des petits ruminants (PPR), is a contagious disease affecting goats and sheep.

Rabies: Rabies is a viral disease that causes acute inflammation of the brain in humans and other warm-blooded animals.

Ruminants: An even-toed hoofed mammal that chews the cud bringup from its rumen. The ruminants comprise the cattle, sheep, antelopes, deer, giraffes, and their relatives.

Surveillance: It is monitoring of the activities.

Toxic: Substance which is poisonous.

Vaccine: A vaccine is a biological preparation that provides active acquired immunity to a particular disease.

Veterinary: Concerned or connected with the medical or surgical treatment of animals, especially domestic animals.

Wild Animals: Undomesticated animal species.

Index